# Cause of Death
## The Story of Forensic Science

Frank Smyth first became interested in criminology as a young
reporter in the West Riding of Yorkshire. Moving up to London,
he worked on the magazine *Crimes and Punishment*. His book
*The Detective in Fact and Fiction* was published in 1977, and in 1979
he was co-author, with the unofficial approval of West Riding police,
of a comprehensive account of the search for the 'Yorkshire Ripper'
called *I'm Jack: The Police Hunt for the Yorkshire Ripper*. Other
published works include *Modern Witchcraft*, *Ghosts and Poltergeists*
and, with Michael Jackson, *The English Pub*.

Frank Smyth

# Cause of Death
**The Story of Forensic Science**

with a foreword by Colin Wilson

Pan Books London and Sydney

Acknowledgments
We would like to thank the following for their help and co-operation
in the preparation of this book: Dr R. Williams, Dr B. Culliford and
Dr Anne Priston of the Metropolitan Police Forensic Science Laboratory;
Detective Sergeant Edward Horne; Joe Gaute; Donald Rumbelow;
Sergeant Barry Shaw and Brian and Eunice Innes.

First published 1980 by Orbis Publishing Ltd
This edition published 1982 by Pan Books Ltd,
Cavaye Place, London SW10 9PG
© Orbis Publishing Ltd 1980
ISBN 0 330 26578 4
Printed and bound in Great Britain by
Cox & Wyman Ltd, Reading

# Contents

# Foreword

I suspect that the fascination of murder lies in the excitement of the battle of wits between the policeman and the criminal. It is a matter of sheer drama. Now it may seem an extraordinary thought: but it is only in the past century or so that the *detection* of a crime has played any major part in the drama. Before that, the methods of fixing guilt were crude and practical. You arrested the man (or woman) who was suspected of the murder and tortured him until he confessed. Or you tossed the suspect into a pond: if he floated, he was innocent. Or you dragged him into the presence of the victim, and if the corpse's wounds bled, he was guilty. The question of detection only arose in those rare cases where the authorities had no means of identifying the corpse.

This occurred, for example, in March 1725, when a night-watchman at Horseferry Wharf – on the Thames – discovered a severed head lying on the mud of the foreshore. The head was carefully washed, the hair combed, and then it was stuck on a stake in St Margaret's Churchyard in Westminster, in the hope that someone would recognize it. When the head began to decay, it was placed in a jar of spirit, and exhibited to anyone who thought they might be able to identify it. Eventually, someone wondered whether it might not belong to a carpenter named John Hayes, who had not been seen recently.

The notion of displaying a severed head in a public place strikes us as rather horrifying; yet the modern equivalent of the method is still in use. Even as I write, the British police are preparing to publish photographs of a head that has been modelled in clay on the skull of an unknown man found near Camberley, Surrey. His body was discovered, decomposed, in a water-filled ditch, and anatomists at Manchester University, with knowledge of the victim's basic characteristics, constructed his probable facial features. Photographs of unidentified murder victims are often displayed on posters. This happened, for example, in 1944, when a woman's corpse was found, in a sack, lying in a stream in Luton, Bedfordshire; she had been battered to death, and the face was severely bruised. Nevertheless, it was photographed, and the picture displayed in public places, and flashed on the screen in cinemas. But although it no doubt gave many of the citizens of Luton 'a nasty turn', it brought absolutely no result. The case was solved by more orthodox detection methods.

Since the corpse was nude, police reasoned that the killer must have disposed of the clothes. Rubbish dumps were searched for old clothes; one torn black coat had a dyer's tag; and, when questioned, the dyer was able to send the police to the house of a man named Bertie Manton, whose wife had been absent for four months. According to Manton, she was staying with relatives. All household goods were fingerprinted, and a print found on a pickle jar in the larder identified the corpse as that of Mrs Rene Manton. The evidence of her dentist confirmed it. Manton confessed to striking his wife with a stool in a jealous rage; he was duly sentenced to death (but later reprieved).

Oddly enough, Mrs Manton's 17-year-old daughter had seen the post-mortem photograph of her mother on several occasions in the cinema, but had failed to recognize it – which might indicate that, in some respects, the methods of the eighteenth century were no less efficient. A severed head is easier to recognize than a photograph.

What Frank Smyth tells in this book is a small but fascinating part of the long battle between civilization and crime. For this is what it really amounts to – not simply a battle between the criminal and the law. If, for example, you consult Luke Owen Pike's *History of Crime in England* (1873), you will find that in 1348, the year before the Black Death reached England, there was literally a state of war between 'organized crime' and the rest of society. Bands of brigands wandered round openly, just as in the Wild West in the days of Jesse James. They attacked lonely houses and set them on fire; they waylaid and murdered travellers; they seized householders and held them for ransom.

There were so many robbers that they would even band together to swarm into a town when a fair was in progress (and the citizens would feel themselves perfectly secure in a crowd), and plunder and kill as they felt inclined. In 1348, Bristol was actually in the hands of a brigand, who treated the town as his own, and seized all the ships in the harbour. And, as Pike makes clear, the criminals were not always illiterate ruffians; they were often the very people who should have been upholding the law. A band of men – including two abbots and many knights – invaded the estate of the Countess of Lincoln, killed all the game, and cut down all the timber. Another band of marauders, including knights and churchmen, invaded the land of the Archbishop of Canterbury, and carried off all his animals, corn and timber. Clearly, this was a time in which no one can have felt much security.

All this is the necessary preface for Frank Smyth's account of the birth of scientific crime detection. For there was really not a great deal of point in scientific detection when crime was so common and so brutal. The necessary precondition for scientific detection is a law-abiding society, where the chief concern of the criminal is not to be found out. As far as England is concerned, the great change began in the year 1748, when the novelist Henry Fielding became a magistrate. Fielding had a new and startling approach to crime. He asked: why not drop the emphasis on barbaric punishments – gibbets and torture chambers – and attempt to *prevent* crime in advance by having an efficient police force? As a result of this approach, the Bow Street Runners were formed, the predecessors of the 'bobbies' of the nineteenth century. And when policemen finally became an established part of the British scene, the great crime wave came to an end. Now, at last, it was the time for the 'detective'.

The actual word 'detective' was invented by Charles Dickens; Tulkinghorn in *Bleak House* introduces Inspector Bucket as 'a detective officer'. That was in 1852, and by that time, the first great 'detective' of fiction, Poe's Dupin, had been in existence more than ten years. Nowadays, it is difficult for us to realize what a piece of sheer inspiration is represented by Dupin. America was still in the midst of the era of lawless violence – like England a century earlier. No 'classic' modern mysteries; just

9

death by violence. (Even the famous Mary Rogers case – which Poe turned into 'The Mystery of Marie Roget' – is not a true murder mystery; subsequent research has revealed that the pretty cigar girl was in the habit of getting herself pregnant and having abortions; she died when one of these abortions went wrong.) So Poe's invention of a detective who solves his cases by reasoning – in the year 1840 – almost amounts to precognition of the future. Two decades were to pass – by which time Poe had been long in his grave – before the first real 'detective' case in British criminal history, the 'mystery of Road Hill House'.

This began on the morning of 30 June 1860, when the nurse-maid of the Kent family discovered that four-year-old Francis Kent was missing from his cot; shortly afterwards, the child's body was found stuffed down a lavatory in the garden, the throat cut from ear to ear. The local police superintendent found himself out of his depth; he arrested the nurse, but soon had to release her for lack of evidence. A man from Scotland Yard – Inspector Jonathan Whicher – was called in. He had the advant-age of being a stranger; unlike his predecessor, he was not overawed by the upper middle-class status of the Kent family in the community. His professional instinct quickly led him to decide that the likeliest candidate for the murder was the daughter of the house, 16-year-old Constance. Constance was the step-sister of the murdered child; her father had married her governess not long after the death of his wife. Constance was jealous, resentful, and had once run away from home, disguised as a boy. A year before the murder, when the child Francis was ill, he was found one morning completely uncovered in his cot, with his socks removed. Someone had made an attempt to give him pneumonia – and Constance was the only member of the family at home at the time.

Whicher arrested Constance; but the evidence against her was purely circumstantial – mainly some question about the disap-pearance of a blood-stained nightdress – and she was released. But five years later, Whicher's instinct was vindicated when Constance confessed to the crime – under the influence of a clergyman – and was sent for trial. She spent the next thirty years of her life in prison.

An interesting footnote has been added to this case by Bernard

Taylor in his book *Cruelly Murdered*. Taylor is convinced – and he backs his theory with sound reasoning – that it was Constance's father who cut the child's throat. He believes that Samuel Kent was having an affair with the nursemaid, and that they were in bed in another room when Constance crept into the nursery and found her step-brother alone. Constance suffocated him, and later stabbed him rather inexpertly, inflicting a wound in his side. She carried the body outside to the lavatory. The nursemaid, entering the nursery soon after, discovered that the child was missing, and told Samuel Kent. He must at first have supposed that his wife (whom he had seduced when she was governess, and his previous wife was still alive) had discovered his absence, and taken the child into her bed. When he realized his wife was still fast asleep, he made a search and found his son's body.

But what could he *do* about it ? If he raised the alarm, people would want to know how he found out that the child was missing so early, and his affair with the nurse would come to light. If his daughter was arrested as a murderer, there would be a double scandal and his career would be ruined.

But there had been a number of murders in the area in recent years – unsolved murders in which the victims had their throats cut. If the child was found with his throat cut, the unknown murderer might be blamed. So, according to Mr Taylor, Samuel Kent fetched a carving knife and cut the throat of the 'corpse'. (In fact, the child may well have been alive.) Then he went back to bed.

Perhaps the oddest footnote to the case is that Constance Kent lived to be a hundred, and died as recently as 1944 in Sydney, Australia, having led a blameless existence as a nurse for more than half a century.

From our point of view, the most interesting point about the Road Hill House mystery is that it brought Inspector Whicher to the attention of such literary men as Dickens and Wilkie Collins, and that Collins transformed Whicher into Sergeant Cuff, the detective-hero of *The Moonstone*. Cuff is generally agreed to be the first real detective in modern fiction (since Dupin was an amateur). Cuff is by no means as brilliant as Sherlock Holmes or some of his later descendants; but he is, in all essentials, the modern policeman who uses all his experience and common-sense in the investigation of a crime.

By the time Cuff made his appearance, in 1868, the 'great age' of Victorian crime was getting into its stride; Mrs Manning, William Palmer, Madeleine Smith, Dr Smethurst, Constance Kent, Franz Muller (the first train murderers) and Dr Pritchard had already been tried; the Wainwrights, the Stauntons, Florence Bravo, Kate Webster, Charlie Peace, Dr Lamson, Adelaide Bartlett, Florence Maybrick, Neill Cream and A. J. Monson were still to come. And, as Frank Smyth here recounts, scientific crime detection at last made its appearance, ushered in by the great Alphonse Bertillon.

This is a name that causes all students of criminology to raise their hats. It is true that Bertillon is now greatly underrated, because his complicated system of criminal measurements was made redundant by fingerprinting. (I have even met criminologists who thought he was the inventor of fingerprinting.) But that is not the point. The point is that Bertillon was the man who brought a new *spirit* to criminology. Before he arrived on the scene, crime was still regarded as a gruesome accident, an act of God, to which the correct response was to get somebody to confess, and then punish him as nastily as possible. In other words, it produced a sense of rage and helplessness. Bertillon declined to share this defeatist attitude. He felt that all crime should be detectable, provided the method was sufficiently scientific. After Bertillon, it was the beginning of a new age – the age which is the subject of this excellent book.

But before I leave the story to Frank Smyth, I feel that I must, in all fairness, acknowledge the crucial role of the French in crime fighting, even before the coming of the 'new age'. England brought the great crime wave to an end with the formation of the police force. The French went further than that; they attempted to bring method to the art of detection. Faced with a crime wave in 1810, the head of the newly founded Sûreté, Henri, conceived the masterly plan of appointing a daring criminal, Eugene Vidocq, his right hand man. Vidocq proved to be a master detective as well as a master criminal, and the story of his exploits is one of the most exciting and astonishing chapters of modern criminal history. Vidocq taught the Parisian police to put themselves in the shoes of the criminal, and to track him through the use of intelligence rather than foot-slogging. Although, in many cases, the two were inseparable.

Perhaps the greatest single piece of detection of those early days must be credited to a young policeman named Gustave Macé, who displayed some of the qualities of Poe's Dupin. In January 1869, a restaurant owner in Paris saw a parcel floating in his well; it proved to contain the lower part of a human leg. Macé was called in, and he soon found another parcel containing a portion of a leg. This was sewed in back calico, and the stitches had a professional look. Macé concluded that the man he was looking for was probably a tailor.

A medical man declared that the legs were those of a woman. Macé spent weeks tracing no less than eighty-four missing women, and finally eliminated every one of them. But his researches had turned up a few more clues. In the previous December, a man had been seen scattering chunks of meat in the river; he explained to a passer-by he was baiting it for fish. Shortly afterwards, detectives had seen a man walking near the river with a hamper; they questioned him, but the man convinced them he had only just arrived in Paris by train, and he looked so honest they let him go. The description tallied; both the meat-scatterer and the man with the hamper were short, dapper men with a black moustache and confident manner.

Why had the man chosen to dump the legs in the well of the restuarant? It sounded as if he knew the house well. Macé asked the concierge if there had ever been a tailor in the house; she said no – but there had been a tailoress. A disappointing lead, but Macé followed it up. For whom did the girl work? Various people, said the old lady; other tailors used to give her work. One of these used to cause problems by spilling water on the stairs, water from the well. Macé traced the tailoress, who told him that the man who used to spill water was called Pierre Voirbo. He had been her lover, but was now married. His description corresponded to that of the man with the basket of raw meat.

By this time, another doctor had stated authoritatively that the legs were not those of a woman, but of an old man. Macé asked the girl if Voirbo had any special friends; she mentioned

13

an old miser named Desiré Bodasse. She had no idea of his address. More foot-slogging brought Macé to Bodasse's apartment. The concierge said she had not seen him for weeks, but was sure he was at home – she had seen a light in his room. But he never answered the door.

Bodasse's aunt was taken to examine the legs in the morgue; a distinctive scar left her in no doubt that they belonged to her nephew Desiré. Macé broke into Bodasse's apartment. Everything was tidy, but a strong box was empty. Macé found a list of the securities it was supposed to contain; but the securities had vanished.

Voirbo was apparently a police spy. This was a period when anarchist bombs frequently exploded in France; Voirbo used to pose as a revolutionary, and make speeches at anarchist meetings; then he would report back to the police. Macé set two of his men to watch Voirbo's apartment. Unfortunately, they recognized him as a 'colleague', and asked him what was going on; Macé's quarry was alerted.

Macé now decided to approach Voirbo direct. Voirbo was apparently eager to help. He told Macé that he was fairly certain that Bodasse had been murdered, and that he, Voirbo, suspected a butcher named Rifer of the crime. Rifer was an alcoholic. And when Voirbo began encouraging him to drink heavily, there was nothing Macé could do. One night Rifer had a fit of DTs, and had to be dragged off to an asylum, where he died.

And at this point, when it looked as if Voirbo had won, Macé decided to arrest him. He discovered he was only just in time; Voirbo had a ticket to America in his pocket.

Macé searched Voirbo's apartment; he found the missing securities soldered into a tin box and suspended in a cask of wine. But he still needed proof that Voirbo had murdered Bodasse. He interviewed the young couple who now lived in Voirbo's old apartment, and asked them about the arrangement of the furniture when they first came to look at it. It soon became clear that, if Voirbo had killed Bodasse there, it would have had to be in the centre of the room, where a table had stood. He had probably been dismemebered on the table. The floor showed no trace of blood; but Voirbo's former landlord described how Voirbo had carefully scrubbed and cleaned the room one morning; he explained that he had spilt a bottle of cleaning fluid on the floor, and that it smelt so much that he decided to scrub the place out.

With fine dramatic instinct, Macé decided to stage the grand finale in this room. Voirbo was taken there, and stood silent, apparently unshakeable. Macé then said: 'If Bodasse was killed here, his blood must have flowed on the floor. I shall now pour water to try to get an idea of how the blood ran.' He tilted a jug; the water ran into a depression under the table. By now, Voirbo was tense and nervous. A mason removed the tiles; the underside was caked with dried blood. Voirbo's nerve gave way, and he made a full confession to the murder. He had asked Bodasse to lend him 10,000 francs, which he needed to marry a girl who would bring him a dowry; Bodasse refused, and Voirbo decided to kill him. He invited him to his room for a cup of tea, then struck him a tremendous blow with a flat iron. After this, he cut his throat, and dismembered the body. Then the remains were thrown in the river – except the legs. Afraid of meeting again the two constables who had already questioned him about the hamper, Voirbo decided to throw the legs into the well of the restaurant.

He made two mistakes. One was to sew the legs up so neatly that Macé guessed that he was dealing with a tailor. The other was to lose his nerve when Macé revealed the dried blood under the tiles. For in 1869, there was no test to distinguish animal from human blood. When Dr Watson first met Sherlock Holmes, some twenty years later, Holmes told him he had just discovered an infallible test for detecting human blood stains; but this was fiction. The actual discovery took place in the year 1900, when Paul Uhlenhuth discovered the interesting properties of blood serum.

But that is part of the story of the 'new age' of crime detection, which is recounted so absorbingly by Frank Smyth in the following pages.

C.W.

# Chapter One
# Science and the law

Whatever the value to society of the advances in
forensic science and, in particular, forensic
medicine, it has provided me with a life of
infinite variety of human interest.

Sir Sydney Smith, *Mostly Murder*

The rural township of Henley, which lies on the banks of the
river Thames in Buckinghamshire, is a peaceful spot noted
chiefly for its annual regatta, during which young men in straw
hats and blazers ply demurely clad ladies with strawberries and
champagne while watching the rowers toil in the mild English
sunshine. If murder were ever to be committed in Henley it
would have to be choreographed, one would think, by Agatha
Christie.

In June 1978, however, Thames Valley police were convinced
that they had a brutal killing on their hands quite uncharacter-
istic of the idyllic nature of the place, although the manner of its
discovery was worthy of detective fiction.

One morning Michael Crossland, landlord of the Drovers
Inn at South End Common, near Henley, went out to feed his
pet goat Henry and found the animal chewing on an old sports
jacket. Mr Crossland retrieved the garment and to his horror
found that it seemed to be covered in blood. He called the police.
Senior officers converged on the pub and examined the coat,
confirming his findings; there was a large hole in the breast
pocket surrounded by what appeared to be powder burns and
the red-brown stains of a massive shotgun wound. Eight policemen and a tracker dog searched the pub grounds, while police
frogmen were despatched to a nearby pond, and the officers of
three neighbouring counties were alerted. By mid-day, telex
messages had widened the dragnet to involve every police station
in the south of England, and hospitals were warned to watch out
for an injured man, on the off-chance that the victim had survived.

Meanwhile the jacket was despatched to a forensic science laboratory, where experts were asked to check on the stains. By the end of the day they had a full story of the 'murder' – to the acute embarrassment of the police. The hole had been made by acid from a car battery, which had reacted with dye in the material and turned brownish-red; experiments showed that in all likelihood some motorist had worn the jacket while leaning over his battery to work on it, and had probably discarded the damaged coat afterwards.

A Thames Valley police spokesman told the press: 'We were convinced that it was blood and we were also sure that it was a bullet hole. This is a very unusual case.'

Ten years previously, according to an article in *The Times*, an equally outlandish case had occurred not far from Henley.

Three little flying saucers were discovered . . . the Army promptly blew one up and the police lost the second down a drain while trying to find out what it was.

The saucers might have become an important chapter in the long history of unidentified flying objects, notwithstanding that drastic treatment, but for the work of a forensic scientist who got to the third before it went the way of its fellows. He discovered it was of glass fibre and an ingenious hoax.

The day-to-day work of the forensic scientist is rarely so sensational, but the two cases do serve to illustrate one important aspect of his function: he reduces hearsay evidence, speculation and theory to bald scientific fact. He is not partisan; in the free world at least, his evidence is available to prosecution and defence counsel alike. He deals in the truth as he and his instruments find it.

The word 'forensic' is frequently misused by the press, police and public alike; it has a Latin root and simply means 'of the courts'. (In this respect it resembles that other popular pseudo-criminological word 'alibi'; this means 'elsewhere' so that logically speaking a suspected person does not have 'an alibi' he 'pleads alibi'.)

To the average member of the public, the word 'forensic' conjures up pictures of a man in a bloodstained apron digging bullets from a dead body while grim-faced policemen look on, and to the extent that the medical branch of forensic science is the largest and certainly the oldest, the concept is a true one. Forensic medicine, or medical jurisprudence, as it is known in the English-speaking countries – the French and Germans use the terms *médecine légale* and *gerichtliche Medizin* respectively – is almost a discipline of its own, but the field is far broader as a whole and is rather less dramatic. Half the work of the world's forensic science laboratories today has been estimated to involve drunken driving cases and road accidents, while another large proportion deals with civil cases such as questions of paternity or industrial accidents. The criminal work, with which this book deals, is relatively small, in proportion to the rest. Nevertheless in 1978 the seven British regional forensic science laboratories (for example) dealt with over 50,000 major criminal cases, in almost all of them achieving success. Increasingly, the dedication of forensic scientists ensures that crime pays less and less.

The principle behind all forensic science cases is a relatively simple one – in theory at least. It was first propounded at the turn of the century by Professor Edmund Locard of Lyons University in the phrase 'every contact leaves a trace', implying that a criminal always leaves something at the scene of his crime and, conversely, takes something away with him. A murderer may leave a body and take away a splash of his victim's blood, a rapist may unwittingly carry off a pubic hair on his clothing while leaving semen stains behind, a hit and run driver may scrape off a flake of paint and carry samples of gravel in his tyre treads. All these things – stains, fingerprints, weapons and bullets, scraps of clothing and fibre – are grist to the mill of forensic science.

Despite its present-day efficiency, forensic science as a regular practical discipline is less than a hundred years old, although in empirical form it has existed for centuries. One writer has quoted King Solomon's judgment on the parentage of a child, when two 'mothers' claimed it, as the first recorded instance of forensic science in action, and the notion is not as fanciful as it may first appear. Modern forensic psychologists would agree with his treatment of the case; it will be remembered that the King called for a sword and offered to cut the child in two, giving half to each claimant; the real mother preferred to let the child live with her rival rather than have it suffer this fate, thus revealing to Solomon her true emotions. Solomon, renowned for his wisdom, was showing his insight into the mind and motive of the criminal.

The first autopsy, a post-mortem examination of a dead body, is attributed to two Alexandrian surgeons, Herophilus and Erasistratus, in the third century BC. They are reported to have carried out dissections for the study of disease, but do not seem to have applied the principle to the examination of murder victims. This 'first' is claimed for the Roman Antistius, who is said to have performed a rudimentary examination of the corpse

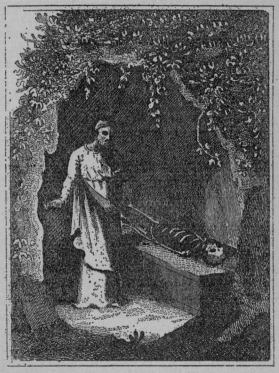

*A romanticized eighteenth-century view of Galen, the Roman physician whose researches entitle him to be known as the first pathologist. (Mansell Collection).*

of Julius Ceasar. He noted 23 stab wounds, and announced that only one – through the heart – had been fatal.

Most authorities, however, claim that the Graeco-Roman physician Galen was the first true forensic pathologist. Certainly Galen, who flourished between AD 130 and 200, performed a number of autopsies, and was the first physician to correlate a patient's external symptoms with the interior signs in his body after death. But his ideas were curious, to say the least. He quotes with approval the case of a fellow doctor who saved a woman from punishment for adultery. The woman bore a child who looked so unlike her husband that the poor man pressed charges against her, adultery being punishable by death at that time. The doctor was called in, examined the woman's bedroom, and pronounced that the child took his appearance from a statue that stood by the mother's bed; she had, he said, looked on it too frequently during her pregnancy, and had thus affected her unborn baby's features.

Many hundred of years were to pass before much further progress in the examination of 'suspect' corpses was made, and even then the development was unknown to the western world. In 1248 an enormous tome entitled *Hsi Yüan Lu* appeared in China, detailing methods of examining murder and assault victims with a view to bringing criminal charges against those responsible. From a general medical point of view the book is important because it seems to predate Harvey by several centuries in suggesting that the blood circulates in the body; from the point of view of forensic science it also made a valuable point, warning its users that 'everything may depend upon the difference between two hairs'.

Like most ancient works on medicine, much of the content of the *Hsi Yüan Lu* was highly speculative, and some of it dealt with out-and-out magic or superstition, but it describes fairly accurate methods of telling whether drowning or strangulation had taken place, what kind of weapon had been used for stabbing the victim, and whether or not a body found in water or burned had been killed beforehand. It also echoes the words of modern police instructors in stressing that the body should be carefully examined at the scene of the crime along with its surroundings.

The *Hsi Yüan Lu* obviously represents a compilation of the

experience of many generations; in Europe, progress was much slower, and it was only in the thirteenth century that the courts of northern Italy first appointed medical experts to advise them. Post-mortem examinations were allowed, particularly in cases of suspected poisoning, but the Church was strongly opposed to anatomical dissection, and it was a brave man who would risk persecution by performing an autopsy on a human corpse. Mondino dei Liucci of Bologna is generally credited with having performed the first public dissection in 1312, but it was not until the publication of the *Humani Corporis Fabrica* of Andreas Vesalius in 1543 that the tide of prejudice turned.

This magnificently illustrated treatise on the structure of the human body has rightly been acknowledged as the foundation of modern medicine. Indeed, five years after its publication Pope Clement VI was actually ordering his personal physician, Guy de Chauliac, to perform autopsies on plague victims in the forlorn hope of discovering a cure for the disease.

In spite of the Church's opposition to human dissection, by the beginning of the sixteenth century the procedure for presenting medical evidence in the law court had been laid down. Concerned about a rise in crimes involving bodily injury and infanticide, the Bishop of Bamberg ordered the compilation and publication of the *Constitutio Bambergensis Criminalis* in 1507; this proposed, among other matters, that a physician be called to any case involving violence to take notes on the nature and position of wounds and draw conclusions from them to be presented in court. In 1516 the Elector of Brandenburg followed suit with a similar publication of his own, which led, in 1533, to the publication of a huge penal code entitled *Constitutio Criminalis Carolina*.

Drawn up by order of Emperor Charles V, it set out codes of legal conduct for the vast tract of central Europe which was the Emperor's domain; despite its fame, however, the book was scarcely an inspiration to potential forensic pathologists of the time. It concerned itself largely with guidelines to physicians in establishing whether or not an accused person was strong enough to be put to torture, and it made little mention of post-mortem examination, except to suggest that wounds should be 'widened' and plumbed to determine the direction and depth of the weapon's penetration.

21

The work of three men, Ambroise Paré of Paris, Fortunato Fidelis of Palermo, and Paolo Zacchia of Rome, marked the major advances of sixteenth-century forensic medicine. All of them were disciples of Vesalius, and took his work a stage further. Paré made a particular study of the vital organs of murder victims – the heart, liver, lungs and so on – and produced a precise description of the lungs of suffocated children; he also described various sex crimes and their visible effects. Fidelis devoted much of his research to drowning cases, detailing them in copious notes, while Zacchia cast his net more shallowly but wider in observing bullet wounds, knife cuts, various forms of asphyxiation, abortion and infanticide, suicide as distinct from homicide, and the effects of certain mental aberrations.

By the end of the century, Theophile Bonet of Geneva had finally vanquished the distaste felt for post-mortem examination by performing around 3000 autopsies and publishing his findings, and he was followed in the first half of the following century by Giovanni Morgagni, usually known as 'the father of modern pathology', who instituted a system of carefully describing, during a post-mortem examination, what could be seen with the naked eye. In 1663, almost contemporaneously with Morgagni, the Danish surgeon Thomas Bartholinus devised what must be one of the first 'scientific' tests in forensic medicine. He announced that the only method of telling whether or not a child had been born alive was to examine the lungs for air; if the child had breathed, then it had been born alive and the corpse must be treated with suspicion. Twenty years later a Doctor Schreyer of Pressburg (now Bratislava) came up with a simple experiment to determine the presence of air in childrens' lungs. He dropped the organs in water; if they floated, air was present.

At this time the atmosphere surrounding pathology was becoming much less rarified, so much so that in 1642 two German doctors, Bohn and Michaelis, began a course in primitive forensic medicine at the University of Leipzig. This was a vital development, bestowing academic respectability on the previously despised science, and during the rest of the century other major universities, notably those of Prague and Vienna, began courses in what was termed 'public medicine' –

dealing with both medico-legal matters and public hygiene.

The concept of 'public medicine' was largely a product of the French Revolution and was perhaps best summed up by the French physician Fodere in 1796, in his *Traité de médecine légale et d'hygiène publique*. This was echoed by a similar publication, the work of the Viennese Johann Peter Franck, at around the same time, and both stressed two basic problems then facing European society: on the one hand, the need for properly qualified medical men to advise the law courts on matters of murder, rape, and injury, and on the other the need to cut down on the epidemics of sickness which stemmed from the concentration of large numbers of people in virtually medieval cities, lacking adequate drainage and water supplies. The *Code Napoleon*, published in 1808, gave administrative flesh to the theories of Fodere and Franck, principally in abolishing torture and throwing open the procedures of European courts for public examination; the work of the 'medical examiner' was thus revealed, not as a secret, ghoulish ritual conducted out of macabre curiosity, but as a vital public service. A 'police surgeon' system was set up, and for many years – far into the nineteenth century – police surgeons could only hold office after having undergone rigorous training at either Prague or Vienna.

Across the English Channel, advances were slow. In 1801, Andrew Duncan, a physician and academic, began lecturing on legal medicine at Edinburgh University. Like his fellow surgeons, however, he was hampered by the laws which restricted the use of bodies for dissection; this in turn led to the heyday of the 'body snatchers' or 'resurrection men' as they were termed. Two of these, Burke and Hare, later became infamous for murdering victims in order to collect money from the medical school at Edinburgh University. Nevertheless in 1807 Duncan had pressed the advantages of European-style 'public medicine' home so thoroughly that his son, also named Andrew Duncan, became Edinburgh's first Professor of Forensic Medicine, holding his post by Crown Commission.

The influence of Europe and Edinburgh had crossed the Atlantic by 1804, when the surgeon James S. Stringham gave a course of lectures at Columbia College, New York, and was so successful that in 1813 he was appointed to the Chair of Medical

# AUTHENTIC
# CONFESSIONS
OF
# WILLIAM BURK,

Who was Executed at Edinburgh, on 28th January
1829, for Murder, emited before the Sheriff-
Substitute of Edinburgh, the Rev. Mr Reid,
Catholic Priest, and others, in the Jail, on 3d
and 22d January.

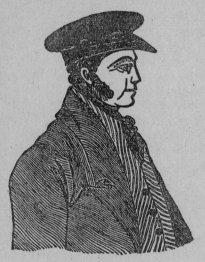

EDINBURGH ：

*Printed and Sold by R. Menzies, Lawnmarket.*

———

## 1829.

*Price Twopence.*

*The most famous of the body snatchers, William Burke, who*
*was hanged for murdering victims to supply Edinburgh's*
*anatomy school. (Radio Times Hulton Picture Library).*

Jurisprudence, instituted by the American College of Physicians and Surgeons in New York City – the first Professorship of its kind in the United States. Under his encouragement, Dr T. R. Beck gave a series of lectures during the same year at the College of Physicians and Surgeons for the Western District at Fairfield, New York. Gradually, over the next few decades, forensic establishments were set up in all the major American medical schools.

Although all this appeared to be progress – and was, of course, compared with the hostility of previous centuries – medicine was in the doldrums. The techniques of anatomical dissection had changed little since the era of Vesalius, and observation was still made largely by the naked eye. It was the widespread use of the microscope – invented in the seventeenth century, but (unaccountably) almost ignored by medical men for more than a hundred years – which altered the pattern of things. The discovery of the cell as the basis for all organic structures, and experiments in microscopic histology – study of the tissues – which led to greater knowledge of the body's make-up, inspired three great contemporaries to set the course of forensic medicine in the modern world.

Mathieu Joseph Bonaventure Orfila, born in Minorca in 1787, arrived in Paris at the beginning of the nineteenth century and began experimenting with and cataloguing poisons and their effects; Orfila was undoubtedly the founder of modern forensic toxicology. His colleague at the University was Marie Guillaume Alphonse Devergie, the man who brought the microscope to bear on practical forensic pathology and produced, in 1835, his classic *Medecine légale théorique et pratique*. Meanwhile, in Berlin, Johann Ludwig Casper, born in that city a year before Orfila, was at work in the pestilential morgue of the *Anatomie*, a building which had changed in neither efficiency nor standards of hygiene since it was built a hundred years previously. He specialized in the corpses of suicides and murder victims, and produced two of the first real guide books for forensic pathologists, *Gerichtliche Leichenöffnung* (Forensic Dissection) in 1850 and 1856 *Praktisches Handbuch der gerichtlichen Medizin* (Practical Manual of Forensic Medicine). These, in several translations, became standard texts throughout the civilized world.

For the next half century, France remained the leading country in the field of medical jurisprudence, not only through the efforts of Orfila and Devergie at Paris, but also through those of Professor Alexandre Lacassagne in Lyons.

Lacassagne was born in 1844 at Cahors, and attended the Ecole Militaire in Strasbourg, before qualifying as a surgeon. Commissioned as an army surgeon he served in North Africa, and it was perhaps this posting which first set him on the forensic path of medicine. Tattoos were very common in Algeria, both among the natives themselves and the French soldiers, and Lacassagne began to think along the same lines that his countryman, Alphonse Bertillon, was to follow – the value of having some means of identifying convicted criminals for the purpose of establishing a police file. He studied tattoos and discovered that they were virtually ineradicable, subsequently publishing a paper on the subject.

Lacassagne's work with the army had also, naturally, brought many bullet wounds to his professional attention, and he began to note the size, shape and appearance of these and other wounds. When he left the service he published the results of his experiences in *Précis de médecine* in 1878, a book which was such a success that when, two years later, it was decided to establish a chair of forensic medicine at Lyons University he was invited to be the first Professor. Lacassagne went on to make several valuable contributions to the sum of medico-legal knowledge. Among them were methods of establishing the time of death, and determining whether in fact a person was actually dead. He made the first observations of hypostasis or post-mortem lividity – the purplish staining of a body caused by the blood draining to its lower points – and he also studied rigor mortis and the rate of cooling of a body as a means of establishing time of death. He never took anything for granted, and coined a phrase still taught in forensic science establishments: 'One must know how to doubt.'

Unfortunately, it was doubt which had temporarily turned the public's mind in Britain by the time Lacassagne was established at Lyons. In 1859 Dr Thomas Smethurst was charged with murdering a woman named Isabella Banks with poison. A leading toxicologist examined tissues from the body and declared at the magistrates' hearing of the case that he had found quantities of arsenic in them. However, by the time of the trial proper he was forced to admit that the arsenic had come from an imperfection in his testing equipment; to make matters worse he and two other forensic 'authorities' on medicine wrangled with each other in court. When Dr Smethurst was convicted despite these scenes there was an outcry, with such august organs as the *Lancet* and *The Times* publicly denigrating the toxicology evidence; such was the force of their arguments that the Home Secretary referred the case to an independent body of specialists, with the result that Dr Smethurst was acquitted. The *Dublin Medical Journal* pronounced that the toxicologist had 'brought an amount of disrepute upon his branch of the profession that years will not remove'.

And so it proved. Not until the Crippen case half a century later, in which vital toxicological and pathological evidence helped to bring about a conviction, did the British press or the 'orthodox' medical world view forensic medicine with anything less than suspicion.

The task of smoothing the ruffles caused by the disastrous Smethurst case fell to three brilliant scientists at St Mary's Hospital in Paddington, London. They were Dr (later Sir) William Willcox, Dr A. P. Luff, and Dr A. J. Pepper. In 1899 they were joined by a young medical student whose fame, greater than that of any other single medico-legal expert, was to spread throughout the world in the next half century – Bernard Spilsbury. Spilsbury was taken under the wing of his three seniors when he showed enthusiasm and aptitude for legal medicine; Pepper in particular encouraged his interest in toxicology and histology, and Spilsbury also took a course in bacteriology along with another young man destined for world fame – Alexander Fleming, discoverer of penicillin.

It was purely on his work, and his announcement of its results in court, that Spilsbury's celebrity rested; despite copious notes on every case he ever handled he never wrote the book he promised, which is perhaps one of the major losses to the medico-legal profession. It was he and Pepper who pulled apart the Crippen defence, and after that his voice in a criminal court became so powerful that his critics, with some justification, claimed that just his appearance for the prosecution could sway the balance of a case.

Even his enemies admired Spilsbury's thoroughness at an autopsy. He examined every inch of the body, front and back, before opening it, and his ability to spot tiny clues which no one else could perceive with the naked eye became legendary. Although his sense of smell was slightly impaired, he could literally 'sniff out' crime in a body or at a murder scene. Once, at an exhumation, he bent over the closed coffin, ran his nose along its edge, and pronounced 'Arsenic, gentlemen'. Until Spilsbury's time, forensic science consisted almost entirely of forensic medicine; even toxicology and ballistics were usually left to the doctor. It was Spilsbury who actively encouraged the development of offshoots of his craft — forensic physics and chemistry, for instance. On one occasion he and a laboratory technician were able to prove that the fluorescence under ultra-violet of a medical dressing worn by a man accused of murder was radically different from that produced by a similar piece of dressing found at the scene of the crime, and the man was discharged.

One legacy left to the world by Spilsbury was the invention of the 'murder bag'. In 1924 he was called to the Mahon case, in which the eponymous Mahon had killed a woman named Emily Kaye and cut up her body into small portions, boiling some of them. When Spilsbury arrived at the scene, on the south coast of England, he was horrified to find a local police superintendent handling the dreadful remains with his bare hands. Apart from any health risks to the superintendent, it was possible that evidence might have been destroyed because of this. Making enquiries, Spilsbury found that the police had no special equipment for scene-of-crime examination, and he set to work to make good this lack. Along with Dr Scott Gillett, he evolved what is now known as 'the murder bag' which is kept packed and ready to be taken to any murder scene. It contained such items as rubber gloves, hand lens, tape measure, straight edge ruler, swabs, sample bags, forceps, scissors, scalpel and other instruments which might be called for. The murder bag was subsequently adopted by every police force in the world.

In 1920, after 20 years at St Mary's, Spilsbury moved to St

Bartholomew's, the great London teaching hospital known as 'Bart's', where he lectured on Morbid Anatomy and Histology, and the following year he received a knighthood. It was ironic that Sir Bernard Spilsbury had been fascinated by the problem of suicide throughout his career; in the late 1940s his powers began to fail him and in December 1947 he gassed himself in his laboratory at University College, London, which was then his headquarters.

If Spilsbury achieved world fame for his achievements, they were at least equalled, in a quieter way, by those of a contemporary, Sydney Alfred Smith. Besides being an excellent surgeon and forensic pathologist, Smith was one of those pioneers who examined the possibilities of forensic science in all its aspects – he contributed directly or indirectly to the fields of toxicology, microscopy, and a great deal, as we shall see in a later chapter, to ballistics. Born in New Zealand in 1883, Smith studied chemistry in his native land before arriving at Edinburgh University, where he qualified in medicine. There he came under the influence of Professor Harvey Littlejohn, who held the Chair of Forensic Medicine, and who had in turn been taught by Dr Joseph Bell, whom Arthur Conan Doyle chose as a model for Sherlock Holmes. In fact Smith himself was to be favourably compared with Holmes many times during the course of his career.

He liked to quote Holme's dictum on the three things necessary for success in a detective: the power of observation, the power of deduction, and a wide range of exact knowledge. Smith himself developed all three to a remarkable degree, amassing knowledge not only on medical matters of every description but on such oddities as the way people wore clothes, the attitude and postures of frightened as against angry attackers and their corresponding defenders, the eating habits of people in different parts of the globe, and so on.

In the early 1920s, Smith was appointed medico-legal adviser to the Egyptian Government, and later founded and became first Professor of the Forensic Department at the University of Cairo. To a keen medico-legal man in those early days the appointment was invaluable, for it enabled him to experiment and form his own opinions entirely independently of outside influences. Poisoning was rife in Egypt, and Smith quickly became an expert on toxicology; shooting and other forms of violence were widespread, and Smith collected firearms and bullets, experimenting with them all the time and building his own comparison microscope for the examination of bullets fired from the same gun, at a time when only a handful were in use in America, land of the instrument's invention.

After his Egyptian appointment came to an end, Smith's connection with Edinburgh University made it the leading centre for the study of forensic science in the world; he was appointed Regius Professor of Forensic Medicine in 1928 and served in the post until 1953. For most of the time he was also Dean of the Medical Faculty, and in 1949 received a knighthood for his services. Even after his retirement he remained Emeritus Professor, and was Rector of the University for three years in the fifties, attracting students from all over the world to his brilliantly witty and idosyncratic seminars. His *Textbook of Forensic Medicine*, first published in 1928, went into over a dozen editions, and when he died in May 1969 he was mourned as a man who, perhaps more than any other, had made forensic pathology into not only an acceptable but respectable branch of medical science.

A close contemporary and colleague of Sydney Smith's was Professor John Glaister, of the Department of Forensic Medicine at Glasgow University. Glaister's massive *Medical Jurisprudence and Forensic Toxicology* is the 'bible' of most British, Australian, and American criminal pathologists today, having been in print, constantly revised, since 1902. But Glaister was no mere theoriser: he and Professor J. C. Brash of the Department of Anatomy at Edinburgh were responsible for carrying out the most complex piece of reconstruction work on human tissue yet recorded, during the Buck Ruxton case of 1935.

Between late September and early November of that year, seventy pieces of human remains were found in a gully off the Edinburgh-Moffat Road, and taken to Edinburgh University for examination. Glaister and Brash had the grisly and complicated task of piecing them together. Obviously they were portions of two murder victims, and judging by three breasts and portions of sexual organs they were those of two women. Beyond this the two doctors could not at first venture, for the killer had gone to enormous lengths to avoid their recognition, cutting off strips of fatty tissue and flesh, removing eyes and lips and scattering the portions over a wide area.

The full details of how they achieved their mammoth task were related by the two professors in their book *Medico-Legal Aspects of the Ruxton Case*, which is also required reading now for pathology students. While they were busy in the laboratory, certain newspapers used to wrap parts of one corpse led police to the Lancaster district in the North of England. There they found that Mrs Isabella Ruxton, wife of a Parsee doctor, and her nursemaid Mary Rogerson had been missing since early September. Dr Buck Ruxton, whose real name was Bukhtyar Hakim, could give no satisfactory explanation of their whereabouts. The police obtained a picture of the 29-year-old Mrs Ruxton, and Professor Brash superimposed this over a picture of one of the skulls taken from the same angle; the fit was exact. This was the first time such a procedure had been used, and it impressed the police so much that they arrested Ruxton immediately.

But, to be certain, Glaister and Brash came up with another novel idea. Two left feet in reasonably good states of preservation had been found among the remains. Flexible casts were taken from these, using a mixture of gelatin, glycerin, and zinc oxide, and were inserted into the shoes of the two women. They fitted. Furthermore, Professor Glaister, on examining the drains at Ruxton's house after the doctor's arrest, found blood and tissue which matched those of the corpses. Detective-Lieutenant Hammond of Glasgow CID visited the Ruxton house and took samples of fingerprints with him. Although the hands of the corpses were badly decomposed, so that much of the epidermis and parts of the dermis had disappeared, Hammond had obtained dermal prints from the hands and successfully matched them with prints found at the house – again the first time that such a procedure had been used. Meanwhile Glaister had called in physicists and other experts to help. Several pieces of cotton sheets used to wrap the bodies were examined microscopically and it was shown that not only had they come from the same loom as portions of sheet found on Ruxton's premises, but from the same warp of that loom. The evidence was so conclusive that Ruxton had no chance, despite the eloquence and skill of his celebrated counsel, Norman Birkett. He was hanged.

*Lancaster.*
*14 . 10 35.*

*I killed Mrs Ruxton in a fit of temper because I thought she had been with a man. I was Mad at the time. Mary Rogerson was present at. the time. I had to Kill her.*

*B Ruxton.*

*The signed confession of Dr Buck Ruxton, who was hanged in 1936 for the murder of his wife Isabella and her nursemaid (from The Murderer's Who's Who by J. H. H. Gaute and Robin Odell).*

The Ruxton case is important in that it was perhaps one of the first major cases in which a team of forensic scientists, rather than one man, brought a killer to justice. Since then team work has been more and more the keyword in scientific criminology, and even 'forensic medicine' becomes increasingly subdivided into specialist fields. Besides the pathologist there is the forensic psychiatrist, especially important in cases where an unbalanced or psychopathic 'random' killer is at large. Odontology – the investigation of teeth – is of increasing importance as more and more dental records are kept throughout the world, although as we shall see it is rather a poor relation in the field of forensic medicine. Immunology and serology, the study of blood, sperm, saliva and urine, are of obvious importance, while the disciplines of toxicology and chemistry speak for themselves.

And today ballistics, especially in a country as gun-conscious as the United States, is an entirely separate field, although of course medical examiners work very closely with the ballistics experts, the wound and the bullet causing it being closely related.

As will be explained, the British Home Office has a laboratory system whereby seven regional 'crime labs', co-ordinated from the former nuclear research establishment at Aldermaston, deal with crime throughout the country. In America, the newly favoured 'medical examiner system', described later, is replacing the old coroner system, although the FBI laboratories are perhaps the only 'national' laboratories covering the country as a whole. On the Continent different systems prevail; Vienna, Leipzig, and Berlin medico-legal institutes send out experts to any Continental police force requesting their assistance, while Denmark has recently set up a unique system of its own. The Denmark State Medico-Legal Council consists of three members, each with different medico-legal qualifications; they examine an average of 4000 cases a year, and although it is perhaps too early to judge their success rate, it does so far seem to be a considerable one.

Thus the youthful discipline of forensic science continues to grow and flourish, never remaining static and, as we shall see in the final chapter, expanding its scope with almost every new development of science as a whole.

# Chapter Two
# Corpus delecti

Here's a corpse in the case with a sad swell'd face
And a Medical Crowner's a queer sort of thing!

Rev. Richard Barham, *A Lay of St Gergulphus*

The formalities that must be gone through in the case of death
are not due solely to superstition or mere caution; apart from
the necessity to determine whether the death is a natural one,
suicide, manslaughter or murder, there is also the question of
property owned or administered by the deceased. The office of
coroner is an English invention, and dates from the twelfth
century, a time when, at least in theory, the entire realm was the
property of the king; and the coroner's duties involved not only
adjudicating on matters of violent and suspicious death but on
questions of property ownership. The name derives from *corona*,
meaning crown, and the coroner was second only to the king in
power and dignity. In other countries the law has changed more
drastically with the abolition of the crown, and preliminary
enquiries into death are now commonly dealt with by the police,
but in England and Wales, and in most countries whose judicial
system derives from English law – including the United States –
the office of coroner has survived. In Scotland, his duties are
performed by the procurator fiscal.

Generally, when a dead body is found, the police will automatically call their official 'police surgeon' – usually a local
general practitioner who has had at least a modicum of medico-
legal training – to examine the corpse at the site and make a
preliminary investigation. The police surgeon and the investigating police officer then report their findings to the coroner;
if there is doubt about the death, the coroner may order an
autopsy to be performed by one of several forensic pathologists
appointed by the Home Office.

In the case of a person who dies at home or in hospital, the
medical attendant examines the body and normally issues a
death certificate stating the cause of death; if he does not know

exactly how the person died, or if he finds anything which strikes him as odd about the death, he says so on the certificate and initials the back, to show that he has reported the death to the coroner.

If he has strong doubts he traditionally – and strictly speaking, illegally – withholds the death certificate altogether, and reports the body as an 'uncertified death'. This is the strongest possible warning that in his opinion further investigation is needed.

Originally, the coroner was a man of substance who was considered to be capable of mature judgment on a case without being influenced either way, rather like the modern British lay magistrate. With the passage of time, however, coroners were appointed because of medical or legal qualifications – a requirement embodied in the Coroners Amendment Act 1926 – and ideally they have a grounding in both. Unfortunately this is not the case with the American coroner system, which has come in for increasing criticism in recent years, and seems destined to be superseded by a more rational medical examiner system.

The American coroner system is a relic of the early New England settlements, when the concept of the coroner was taken to the colonies by the puritans. Its early high idealism was soon flawed by corruption, however, particularly in the small communities where self interest on the part of the coroner often entered a case. As opponents of the system point out, the temptation to bribery – if a rarity in fact – is still there today, for the office of coroner in most American states is a political appointment like that of mayor or sheriff, and the potential coroner needs no qualification other than that of eligibility to run on the predominant party ticket. Although some American coroners are doctors or lawyers – Los Angeles, for instance, has a Chief Medical Examiner who is also Coroner – they are in a minority. Almost by tradition, local undertakers or funeral parlour owners are chosen to occupy the post.

When a County election is held – every two to four years – a coroner is appointed and he in turn appoints up to a dozen or more deputies, all of whom are eligible to hear cases. The coroner's office pays the salary of the deputies, as well as those of at least one full-time forensic pathologist, often with an assistant who specializes in, say, toxicology or ballistics, and a

35

handful of part-time doctors who are not required to have any medico-legal training. One of the major flaws in the coroner system is due to this fact: young, newly qualified medics are cheaper to employ as coroner's physicians and are usually eager to get the work, however badly they may bungle it while gaining experience.

Another outstanding flaw, incredible to European pathologists and those who advocate the medical examiner system, is that when the office is informed of a sudden or suspicious death, usually by a funeral parlour, the corpse has often been embalmed by the time the physician arrives to make his examination; in the larger cities, where deaths runs into hundreds a week, this sort of laxity is appallingly commonplace.

The political nature of the coroner's office also interferes with the work of investigation. According to the British criminal pathologist Dr A. Keith Mant, who made a survey of American medico-legal methods in the 1960s, the full-time forensic pathologist for an area, aided by his part-time staff, may carry out up to 2000 autopsies a year, but although the police are usually in favour of him viewing the body at the scene of a crime, the coroner tends to discourage this. If the crime is likely to make headlines, the coroner can make political capital by turning up himself – unqualified as he may be – and gaining valuable publicity. He prefers the more newsworthy forensic examiner to stay in the background.

So it is that when the pathologist first sets eyes on the corpse, it is usually in the mortuary, where the local Homicide Bureau will have undressed it, photographed it, made a note of any wounds or abrasions, and taken fingerprints. The 'missing persons' detective – attached permanently to most city morgues – will be checking his lists, and the crime laboratory detective, from a mobile unit which visits each morgue daily, will be checking the clothes, nail-parings and so on of the victim. The homicide detective gives the pathologist a history of the case, and the pathologist then conducts the autopsy and notes his findings.

Perhaps most disturbing of all is the fact that the pathologist is rarely called to give evidence in the coroner's court; only his report is submitted by the prosecution, and the coroner's juries frequently miss the point without the medical man being present in person to interpret the wounds or other injuries – whether caused by shooting, stabbing, accident or suicide. Here again, the jury is politically appointed at the coroner's discretion and, for major crimes, is picked from influential citizens, known as a 'Blue Ribbon' jury. Again, this is a political device to publicize the coroner personally and gain him extra votes at the next poll.

It was during the crime boom of the 1920s that thinking citizens first began to question the coroner system, which at best was clumsy and incompetent and at worst riddled with corruption. New York City had for some years abolished the coroner and instead paid medical examiners to work shoulder to shoulder with the police Homicide Bureau in investigating murders from the first stage. Then in 1948, the Commonwealth of Virginia set up a state-wide medical examiner system, abolishing the old county-to-county coroner set-up. Under the new system, the medical investigation of death is separated completely from the legal side.

Dr Mant cites the present day Virginia organization as typical of the ideal being aimed at by medico-legal reformers. The office of the Chief Medical Examiner is in the state capital, Richmond, and has close ties with the Medical College of Virginia, also situated in the city. Part of the responsibility of the Chief Medical Examiner is to direct the instruction of students in the Department of Legal Medicine and the Division of Forensic Pathology there – he is chairman of both faculties. As well as the Central Office at Richmond, there are three other offices, directed by a Deputy Chief Medical Examiner, at Norfolk, Roanoake, and Arlington, each of which is equipped with an up-to-date laboratory and technical facilities, and a full staff of forensic pathologists, toxicologists and physicists. To these come the working Medical Examiners with their findings.

Virginia has now more than 350 ordinary 'MEs', usually two to a city or county, who are the nearest equivalent to the British police surgeon. All of them have undergone a course of training in forensic medicine, and when a sudden death occurs they are notified by the police and given total charge of the corpse. Unlike their counterparts under the old coroner's system, they are obliged to examine the body as it lies, and make a full examination of it clothed and unclothed, before questioning anyone relevant to the death – relatives, friends, personal physicians and hospital staff. With this mass of information at hand they then make their reports to the office of the Chief Medical Examiner and he either issues a death certificate or orders an autopsy.

Autopsies are always carried out by the Chief ME or one of his deputies, the equivalent of the British Home Office-appointed pathologists; after the autopsy no inquest is held, the examiner merely ticking a box on his report form to indicate whether in his opinion death was due to natural causes, accident, suicide or homicide.

As Dr Mant puts it: 'One advantage of this system is its flexibility. The Medical Examiner's classification of death into natural, suicide or homicide is for statistical purposes, and if at some later time evidence should come to light, for instance, that an accident was suicide, or a natural death a homicide, he merely informs the Registrar of Deaths. This has obvious advantages over the lengthy procedure necessary to change a Coroner's verdict in Great Britain.'

The role of the ordinary medical examiner in the United States, and his equivalent the police surgeon in other countries, in the investigation of murder is at least as important as that of both the pathologist who will conduct the autopsy and the senior detective in charge. Indeed to some extent he must anticipate all their roles, as did one astute ME in a case quoted by Dr W. G. Eckert to the American based International Reference Organization in Forensic Medicine.

On a recent case in the United States involving the murderer of several prominent people, the medico-legal investigator called upon his colleagues in forensic psychiatry to aid him and the police with their evaluation of the type of individual or individuals who might commit such a crime. In this regard the total picture was reviewed, including the character and activities of the victims, their environment and behaviour before the crime. The resulting report bore a very astute number of observations and opinions of the type of murderer or murderers who might be involved, and as the alleged murderers were apprehended their character and behavioural pattern fitted very nicely into that which the psychiatrists had predicted. This approach may be unique and non-applicable to most cases, but it does offer a very useful and helpful approach in those cases where the picture is very strange and little evidence is left at the scene.

But for all the triumphs attributable to the police surgeon in the field, as it were, there must be failures – sometimes disasters – and in fact the whole area of medico-legal investigation is riddled with potential pitfalls. In 1956 Dr Alan Moritz presented his address 'Classic Mistakes in Forensic Pathology' which has become itself a classic text for students and aspiring police surgeons. He listed no less than 14 basic mistakes which occur all too frequently where the police surgeon has insufficient experience or acts too hastily; they include performing an incomplete autopsy, permitting the body to be embalmed before a medico-legal autopsy, regarding a mutilated or decomposed body as unsuitable for autopsy, failing to recognize or misinterpreting post-mortem changes, failing to make an adequate examination and description of external abnormalities, not examining the body at the scene of the crime, not taking adequate photographs, and 'talking too soon, too much, or to the wrong people'.

The penultimate complaint may well become a thing of the past with the introduction of video-taping of the body *in situ*. This advance was introduced first by the brilliant Dr Thomas T. Noguchi, Chief Medical Examiner to Los Angeles, and the man who carried out the investigation and autopsy on Robert Kennedy. But the last fault is a frequent one, and is constantly stressed by pathology lecturers to their students, as is the need for constant percipience – close observation of what is there to be seen.

Dr Keith Simpson recalled with horror the spectacle which greeted him in the Southwark mortuary in 1934. A local doctor acting as police surgeon – completely without special training – was leaning against the mortuary wall in his hat and coat, idly making notes as the mortuary keeper – again with no medical training whatsoever – took out and cut up organs from the body of a murder victim. That sort of procedure has, of course, gone for good, but mistakes such as those outlined by Dr Moritz still occur.

Again, Dr Simpson recalled a case in which the police surgeon walked over one body – which no one had yet observed – to examine another. In another case, a woman doctor was called to a house in which a dead man lay slumped in a doorway. She examined the body and left after certifying the fact of death. 'Later in the afternoon a kindly police sergeant rang to ask her if she would mind if he added to her report that "on further examination she found the body to be suspended by a rope attached to the door jamb"!'

In another case in Westminster, a police surgeon removed the plastic bag and ligature which had been tied over the head of a dead child, destroying evidence in the process; the fact that the body was already decomposing meant that everything could have been left as it was without disturbing the scene. Even senior police officers are capable of making such mistakes, as Dr Simpson recalled of a case in Bedfordshire. A girl had been found murdered in a wood, and two policemen arrived on the scene in a squad car. The senior of the two sent his colleague back to the car to radio for an ambulance, and then collected the girl's handbag, shoes and panties, slung her body over his shoulder, and began to walk to the road to help, as he thought, facilitate transport.

Suddenly realising his awful stupidity, he marched back again and laid everything out as – he thought – it had been. A Yard team spent several hours on the scene photographing, recording details – only to have the truth come out when routine checks revealed the fact that the only fingerprint, on the heel of the shoe, was the officer's.

As well as taking things from the scene of death, leaving things there can be equally awkward. The obvious examples are fingerprints and footprints, but there is an amusing story of a Home Office pathologist who left his umbrella, complete with his fingerprints, in the flat of a murdered prostitute, thus causing himself considerable embarrassment.

Ideally, the police surgeon first on the scene of a death obeys a strict pattern of behaviour. If the body is obviously fresh, his first task is, of course, to make sure that it is dead, using his stethoscope and disturbing the clothing as little as possible; if he has to unbutton a shirt or blouse he makes a careful note of what he has done. Today, most police surgeons carry a Polaroid camera to record each stage of their activities. As soon as he knows that the body is dead, he stand back and lets the official police photographers do their work, while as little as possible is disturbed; at this stage he observes the old maxim 'hands in pockets, eyes open, mouth shut'.

It is important that he stays on the scene with the photographers, because he may wish them to record details which will fade or change later – a flow of blood, a drying stain, the angle of a stabbing weapon or the position of a pistol in the hand.

Then, as soon as possible, he begins to take temperature readings. The room or ambient temperature comes first, and then that of the body. Readings from the rectum or vagina are best, but if these are likely to have been interfered with in a sexual attack, the interior of the abdomen is as good. Dr Simpson recommends that a small hole is made, well away from any stab or shot wounds, to take liver readings. The thermometer is inserted into the incision and left for half an hour, and then the hole is sealed with sticking plaster and marked, so that it causes no confusion later.

Throughout the proceedings the police surgeon – like the murder squad detectives, the photographer, and the scene-of-crime fingerprint officers – should take copious notes, with drawings and measurements of anything that may be relevant. Then, while waiting for the pathologist, his final task is to see that the body is not disturbed in any way. Even when the pathologist has made his examination, the undertakers removing the corpse have to be supervised, for careless handling can dislodge hairs or smear blood. Any head wounds are protected by a plastic bag, and the hands – which will later be required for both fingerprints and nail-parings – are similarly protected.

Unless the facts are obvious – in the case of eyewitnesses for instance – the police at this point will turn to the pathologist for immediate assistance in determining the time of death, and he will establish this as far as possible before beginning the actual autopsy. As far as possible, because the condition of a corpse at any given time after death depends on a great number of variables which must all be taken into consideration; but fortunately the time of death can usually be established to within an hour or two.

When death occurs there is an immediate relaxation of the

muscles, which gradually changes over a period of ten to twelve hours into the condition known as rigor mortis. During this period the eyes lose lustre and take on a glazed look, but can be indicative to the pathologist as to time of death. For variable times after death has occurred tissue and molecular activity remain, and if this activity is still continuing, a drop of atrophine on the pupil of the eye will cause it to contract.

Cooling of the body is the main test of death time, although again many considerations have to be taken into account. During the first few hours after death the body cools fairly quickly and then begins to slow down as it approaches the temperature of the surroundings. The limbs cool rather quicker than the main trunk, which is why rectal and liver temperatures are usually taken straight away, or as soon as possible. The surface of the body will generally be completely cold within eight to twelve hours, but complete cooling of a well nourished, clothed adult body will not reach room temperature for 20 to 30 hours. Glaister, in his *Medical Jurisprudence*, suggests a formula to arrive at approximate estimation of the time of death:

$$\frac{\text{(normal temp) } 98.4°F - \text{rectal temp}}{1.5} = \text{approx hours}$$

In Celsius equivalents this formula would be: (37° – rectal temperature) × 1.1 = approx. hours. The average fall in temperature in the first few hours is about one degree F per hour, increasing slightly as time goes on.

But even Glaister's formula is not a hard and fast rule; thin people cool quicker than fat ones, healthy slower than weak, and (obviously) naked bodies quicker than clothed. Bodies cool quicker in water than in air, and if the body is found out of doors allowances have to be made for recent weather conditions. Certain kinds of death – by lightning, electrocution or asphyxia – cause the body to retain heat for a longer period, and in some cases of death by certain diseases – yellow fever, smallpox and cholera, for instance – the temperature may actually rise a little after death.

Next in importance in establishing death time is the presence of hypostasis, or post-mortem lividity, but it has an even more important function in forensic medicine. Hypostasis is the draining of blood to the lowest area of the body when circulation ceases. Within six to eight hours the purplish stains are fixed, but patches of unstained skin are left at the points where the body has been in contact with the surface on which it lies. Because of this it is immediately apparent if a body has been moved after lying for some time in one position. Hypostasis does not occur where pressure has been applied to the surface of the body so that if, for instance, a rope had been tied tightly round the neck, or the body had been bound and the rope or bonds removed some time after death, the marks would show as white marks against the surrounding lividity.

Discoloration is also caused to bodies through various factors – carbon monoxide poisoning, for instance, may leave the victim cherry red, while a similar effect is often produced by hydrocyanic acid or cyanide poisoning. And, of course, lividity on certain parts of the body may be caused by bruising, if violence is suspected. All young forensic pathologists are warned on this point; colour alone is no guide in differentiating hypostasis and bruising. To tell them apart, an incision is made into the centre of the discoloration: if it is hypostasis only a few oozing capilliaries will be noticed, while in the case of bruising blood will have coagulated under the skin.

As well as temperature and post-mortem lividity, the pathologist will use the onset of rigor mortis as a guide to time of death. Rigor mortis is, simply speaking, caused by coagulation of the muscle plasma which tenses and stiffens the muscles in strict order. First to set are the eyelids, about an hour to an hour and a half after death; about an hour to an hour and a half after this the jaw muscles become rigid, and then rigor progresses through the muscles of the neck, the face, the thorax, the arms, the trunk, and finally the legs, and is usually complete after ten to twelve hours. About 36 hours later the rigor mortis passes off, starting with the eyelids and finishing with the feet in the order in which it appeared.

Rigor mortis is often quoted by detective story writers as being the certain test of time of death, and as a rule it is of considerable assistance. Unfortunately, circumstances can alter it enormously. A strong man's muscles will stiffen much later, and remain in rigor for much longer, than those of an old or feeble person. If a body in which rigor mortis is setting in is subjected to a temperature of 75°C, rigor will be completed very rapidly; on the other hand where people have died under icy conditions at or below freezing point, rigor has not appeared at all until the body was removed to warmer conditions. Thus theoretically it would be possible to murder someone and immediately refrigerate the body for purposes of establishing an alibi, say, producing the body later and allowing rigor to be established naturally. A trained forensic pathologist would, however, note changes in the blood and internal organs at the autopsy.

Again, if a person is killed by burning or complete immersion in scalding liquid, a condition resembling rigor mortis immediately comes about and the body remains stiff until the onset of putrefaction.

Another form of rigor, known as cadaveric spasm, is of vital importance where violent death is concerned, and is always noted carefully. Often in cases of suicidal cut throat, or suicidal shooting, the hand holding the weapon is found clutched so tightly around it that it is impossible to disengage it without using considerable force. The condition also occurs in cases of death by drowning, where often the most useless objects are grasped, apparently in an attempt to stay afloat – hence the expression 'clutching at straws'.

As Glaister says: 'This condition is, without question, due initially to a vital voluntary act, probably accompanied by a high degree of emotion, immediately preceding death'.

Most importantly, it is a condition impossible to simulate, so that if the medical examiner finds a weapon or other article clutched in a dead hand in this way he knows that it was in the hand of the person during life and that the grasp occurred at or about the moment of death.

With the fading of rigor mortis, putrefaction of the body sets in, and again there are numerous conditions to be observed to give an estimate of the time of death. Putrefaction begins with the abdomen and spreads outwards to the rest of the body, but is very much dependent on the temperatures and conditions in which the body lies. If the body is dried rapidly, for instance, it may become mummified, or partially mummified, for moisture is the essence of the process. On the other hand, 'it may be accepted as a guiding principle,' says Glaister, 'that a body decomposes in the air twice as quickly as in water, and eight times as rapidly as in earth'.

Young people decay much more quickly than old, because of the relative absence of fat in the latter, and people who die violently in good health resist decay better than those who die of illness. Certain poisons, arsenic, carbolic acid, antimony and zinc chloride, for instance, sometimes preserve the body indefinitely, as in the case of Napoleon Bonaparte related in another chapter; ironically enough, chronic alcoholics may literally be 'pickled' in death, because of the preservative qualities of alcohol.

Once having established the time of death, and satisfied himself that death was due to homicide or other violence, the medical examiner recommends a post-mortem; in America, as we have seen, the Chief Medical Examiner or coroner orders the autopsy; while in Britain the coroner does so, and in Scotland the Procurator Fiscal presents a petition to the local Sheriff. Once a warrant for autopsy is received, the operation is carried out after the formal identification of the dead person by relatives or close friends. In important cases, two medical men may attend, one to do the manual work, the other to take notes and photographs.

First, a thorough external examination is carried out; bruises, cuts, wounds and marks of ligatures are probed, measured, and described. The hands are examined carefully for defensive marks such as knife slashes or broken fingernails; X-ray photographs may be taken of the body at this stage in a search for possible fractures.

The process of internal examination is a lengthy and complex one, if properly carried out, and must include, in the words of Glaister: 'an examination of all the organs of all the cavities of the body, even although the apparent cause of death has been previously found in one of them, since evidence contributory to the cause of death may be found in one or more of the others. The importance of this cannot be too strongly insisted upon, as inadvertent omission of a complete examination may readily invalidate a report.'

A striking instance of what can go wrong if this advice is not followed occurred in Scotland, when a police surgeon was asked to examine a victim of violence. He discovered that there were bruises on the head and chest, but when he examined the heart came to the conclusion that the man had died of a heart attack, probably brought on by the beating. His report was considered unsatisfactory, and a further examination was made; the unfortunate doctor was forced to admit that he had overlooked the fact that the man had a broken neck.

As each organ is removed it is examined and if necessary placed in a glass jar for further tests to be made. Blood and urine samples are taken, and the stomach contents are carefully examined and sent for analysis. The stomach contents are of particular importance, not only in cases of suspected poisoning but also in establishing time of death, in relation to the last meal eaten by the victim. Most meals leave the stomach in about four hours, but a large meal may stay for up to five, and a small meal rich in butter or cream may stay for a longer period. Manufactured carbohydrates such as sugar leave the stomach much more quickly than natural carbohydrates such as potato or banana, and a very fatty meal stays in the stomach perhaps longest of all.

Bruises are usually excised from the body for further examin-

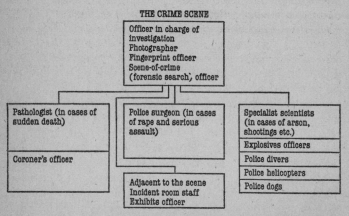

*A chart drawn up by an instructor at the Police Training School shows clearly the inter-relationships of members of the forensic team.*

ation, and sometimes possible identifying marks such as tattoos or old scar tissue – as in the Crippen case detailed later. In the case of carbon monoxide poisoning, separate blood samples are taken from the left and right side of the heart. Swabs are taken from the mouth and, in the case of sexual assault, from the vagina and rectum; in this case pubic hair samples are also taken. Hair is taken from the head in cases of head wounding, and in firearm cases will later be microscopically examined along with scrapings of any powder staining around the entrance wound, in an attempt to establish the range of fire.

Where a body has been burned, mucus is removed from the air passages to determine the presence of carbon particles; if present they indicate that the victim was alive at the time of the burning.

Finally, the notes made during the operation are checked through, the body is closed, and the forensic pathologist makes his report.

Accident, suicide, or murder is what the lengthy report, carefully written for a potential jury in the simplest possible terms, will indicate. If it is murder, the court will require specimens and photographs as well as notes when and if the killer comes to trial, and his defence counsel will also need to see the evidence; for this reason the medical examiner must always be strictly impartial – like all other members of the forensic team who must determine the cause of death.

# Chapter Three

# A question of suicide

Once you are married, there is nothing left for you,
not even suicide, but to be good.

Robert Louis Stevenson, *Virginibus Puerisque*

Late one afternoon in the early 1970s a likeable though
somewhat dowdy blonde named Iris Nina Seagar fell two
hundred feet from the balcony of her Baltimore penthouse to
an abrupt death on the sidewalk below. Making routine inquiries, the Baltimore police department found that Iris had
been popular with her neighbours: admired indeed for the
forebearance with which she tolerated her hard-drinking,
violent husband.

'He was always beating up on her,' said one. 'His drunken
conduct would drive anyone to suicide.'

Iris's husband, the sole eye-witness, claimed, however, that
his wife had not killed herself intentionally. 'She was fiddling
with a faulty air conditioner and tipped over the guard-rail' he
explained. 'I told her not to do it, and said that it was dangerous.'

The police were inclined to leave the matter there, until
insurance officials reported that the husband was the benefici-
ary of Mrs Seagar's $100,000 insurance policy which, naturally
enough, contained a clause nullifying it in the case of suicide.
Suspicious, the Baltimore homicide squad called in a forensic
physicist and a firm of architects. The latter took photographs
of the building from which Iris had fallen from all aspects,
while the former supervised the modelling of several life-like
dummies, simulating the 48-year-old woman's 5 feet 3 inch
figure and 127-lb weight.

A video recorder coupled to a closed circuit camera with
zoom lens was used to record the scene as each dummy was
dropped, thrown, pushed, and tipped over the balcony in an
attempt to reconstruct every possible way in which Iris Seagar

could have died. The VTR tapes were played over and over again so that the trajectories of the falling bodies could be studied, and one glaring fact emerged. A body falling from a high building tumbles outwards for a second or two, and then plummets straight down; the repeated drop tests showed that Mrs Seagar could not have landed more than ten and a half feet from the wall of the building, taking into consideration the architectural features involved, had she fallen accidentally.

In fact she had hit the ground 16 feet 8 inches out into the road. A person cannot jump further in free air than on the ground, and the plump, middle-aged Iris could not possibly have jumped such a distance, even in a determined suicide bid. Faced with this evidence, her husband confessed to throwing her from the balcony in a drunken fit of rage, and was convicted of murder.

In 1959 a handyman named Jackson was found dead in Joplin, Missouri, apparently the victim of homicide. A three-inch wood chisel had been driven into his throat with such violence that it had almost severed the vertebrae of the neck. Jackson had been having an overt affair with another man's wife, and the husband had been heard to threaten him on several occasions; a few nights previous to Jackson's death the two had fought in a bar, and the police had been called. The husband was arrested and, although he pleaded ignorance of the alleged crime, could not provide an alibi. Fortunately for him, however, the medical examiner thought that there was something odd about the angle of the chisel in Jackson's throat; it did not seem likely that an attacker would have struck him in such a way. And in fact fingerprint evidence showed that Jackson had gripped the chisel in both hands and forced it into his own neck, committing suicide in an almost unbelievably vigorous manner.

These two cases illustrate the dangers and pitfalls which may beset police and medico-legal examiners investigating cases of violent death. Casual assumptions, however 'obvious' the facts may seem, can lead to dangerous mistakes being made. Professor Keith Simpson, in a paper for *Criminologist* magazine entitled 'Percipience and the Police Surgeon', observes:

It is often said that the police surgeon at the scene should keep his eyes open, his hands in his pockets, and his mouth shut. In fact, as always, there are exceptions to these good rules. He may with profit "shut his eyes" to some early opinion forming that is so common. "This looks to me like . . ." is often said too early, and what looks at first sight like suicide may, on closer examination, prove to be murder – or the contrary may emerge.

The possibilities of reconstructing events from observation and deduction on the part of the medical examiner are brilliantly demonstrated in a case dealt with by Sir Bernard Spilsbury in May 1911. An insurance clerk named Surgey was found dead in the street in the London borough of Hornsey. His throat had been cut – the exterior jugular vein was completely severed – but a post-mortem showed that he had died of an air-embolism rather than loss of blood. There was a brand new pocket knife, bloodstained, in his right jacket pocket, and in his right hand he clutched a bloodstained handkerchief. His pupils were dilated.

Spilsbury visited the scene of the incident, and pieced together what he was sure must have been Surgey's mental and physical processes. A large splash of blood marked the spot where Surgey had cut his throat, and then isolated stains on the pavement showed how he had walked almost a hundred yards, turned a corner, and collapsed. Spilsbury deduced that, seconds after doing the deed, Surgey was overcome with horror. He had closed the pocket knife, placed it in his pocket, taken out a handkerchief and attempted to staunch the wound; he had then set off to walk to his doctor's house, rather than home, and had turned the corner of the street where the doctor lived before removing the handkerchief for a moment – a large spurt of blood showed the spot where this had occurred – little realizing that by doing so he was letting air into his veins and so determining his death. A few yards further on he had collapsed and died. The pressure of the handkerchief on his neck was such that it had paralysed the sympathetic nerves – showing his belated will to live – and this had caused the pupil dilation.

Such careful reconstruction of events leading up to a suspicious death obviously cannot be expected in the majority of cases. The average police surgeon or medical examiner is a busy man and after all only a minority of cases of what look at first like suicide or accident later turn out to be murder. If he has time a killer will naturally attempt to disguise his work, and there must be countless incidents scattered through history where he has succeeded. Only the failures are known to us.

In the 1930s Sir Sydney Smith was called to the apparently accidental shooting of a drunken Scottish farmer, who was found in a field with his hand on a 12-bore shotgun. The man was married, and he and his wife ran the small farm with the help of a half-witted boy of 15 who lived in an outhouse or 'bothy' in the yard. The farmer had frequently come to the attention of the police because of his drunken rages.

On the day before his body was found, he had gone into a nearby town and spent all evening drinking in the local public house until it closed at 10 pm. Then he had taken a bus back home, and shortly after 11 o'clock, according to the farm boy, had lurched into the 'bothy' demanding that the lad get out of bed and help him shoot 'cushies' (pigeons). The boy had been frightened, and refused. The following morning he had found his employer lying dead in a field, the gun by his side. The farmer's wife claimed to know nothing of all this; she had gone to bed at 10.25 pm, she claimed, and had been aroused by the farm hand the following morning with the news that her husband was dead. She had called the police, and Smith arrived on the scene that afternoon.

The assumption of the police was that the farmer had fallen over and accidentally shot himself, but a cursory examination convinced Smith that this was not so. The body lay face downwards in the long grass, its arms stretched out on either side of the head, about 75 yards from the main farm buildings. A cap was on the back of the head, and when it was removed Smith saw that the scalp was matted with clotted blood, the result of wounds which had not been caused by gunshot. The inside of the cap, however, was hardly stained, which seemed to indicate that it had been placed on the head after the head wounds were inflicted.

In the middle of the farmer's jacket was a huge bloodstain, but no wound tallied with it. Smith pulled the jacket up and found that the bloodstain fitted exactly over the head wound;

he deduced that the jacket must have been in contact with the head wound shortly after it was inflicted, and while it was still bleeding copiously. He soon saw why. The inside of the bottom part of the jacket was stained with earth, grass, and vegetable matter; the shirt and waistcoat were wrinkled up towards the shoulders and had also been smeared with grass and earth stains, and portions of soil adhered to dried bloodstains on the backs of the hands. Almost certainly the body had been dragged along the ground on its back feet first after the head injuries had been received.

The double barrelled 12-bore which lay beside the corpse contained one discharged cartridge in the left hand barrel, the right chamber being empty. On the dead man's left arm was a shotgun wound, and some of the pellets had passed through into the back of the jacket. When the body was rolled over, there was a huge shotgun wound on the left cheek. Smith bent down and examined the wound closely; it had caused massive bleeding, but no signs of blood ran towards the neck area, and the wound's edges were rucked up towards the eye. Again, wrinkling of the clothing towards the head and the presence of grass stains upon it showed that the body had also been dragged feet first on its face for some distance, after the infliction of the gunshot wound to the cheek.

Smith examined the grass surrounding the dead man and quickly spotted a trail of blood leading back towards the farm buildings, which ended in a stackyard, bare of any vegetation, and consisting of trampled earth. One patch looked rather too smooth, and had been tamped down; Smith dug his penknife into the surface and found a large patch of dried blood a couple of inches beneath – so this was the site of the wounding.

Now he had the body removed to his laboratory and performed a post-mortem. The massive loss of blood showed that all the injuries had been inflicted before death, the immediate cause of which was the gunshot wound to the cheekbone, resulting in shock, haemorrhage, and asphyxia due to the inhaling of blood into the lungs; however, the injuries to the scalp had been inflicted first, probably – judging from the shape of the three skull fractures – with the butt end of an axe. They appeared to have been struck from above, and would probably cause un-consciousness instantly.

Examining the shot wound to the face, Smith could see no immediate signs of powder marks, but after removing tissues and examining them under the microscope he found that traces were present; from this and the spread of shot he concluded that the farmer had been shot from a distance of about two yards. The shot that caused the wound to the left arm had been fired from a distance of about three yards, while the victim was lying on his back, and after he had been dragged some distance on his back – exit wounds in the shirt and jacket indicated this.

Smith was now faced with the problem of fixing the probable time of death, a difficult task to be precise about. Rigor mortis had been complete when he first saw the body at 2 pm, and as the rigor process normally takes from ten to twelve hours, death could have taken place between 2 am and 4 am, possibly earlier. The temperature of the corpse at 4 pm, when removed to the laboratory, was 81°F (27°C), so that if it was normal at the time of death it had lost about 17°F (10°C). The atmospheric temper-ature at the time was 68°F (20°C). Again, it is not possible to be certain about the cooling of a body, but Smith reckoned that it would have lost about 8°F in the first four hours and about 1°F per hour subsequently; this gave a calculation of 3 am as the time of death.

Finally, there was the relationship of the alcohol content of the blood and urine. Ordinarily, the two figures are approxi-mately the same, about 1:1.3. In the case of the farmer, the urine contained about three times as much alcohol as did the blood, due to the fact that whereas blood alcohol is gradually diminished through oxidation, that excreted into the bladder alters very little. From this and other physiological factors, Smith calculated that the farmer had lived for about five and a half hours after he stopped drinking, and as the pub closed at 10 pm and there was no evidence of drink around the farm the time of death must have been around 3.30 am.

Now it was a question of filling in the missing four hours between his staggering off the bus and dying; and the relation-ship of the wounds to each other could help there. Death had been caused within minutes by the shotgun wound to the face, but microscopic examination of the scalp wound showed that this had been inflicted about three hours before he died, for leucocytes – white blood cells which flow to the site of a wound to begin the healing process – were discernible.

Smith now began to reconstruct the crime. The farmer arrived home at 11 pm very drunk. He was hit several times by a weapon which resembled an axe, either while he was sitting or when his assailant was at a higher level. Marks of whitewash on his clothes showed that he had been attacked in either the bothy or the farmhouse – both were heavily whitewashed on the inside. He had then been dragged on his back, feet first, into the stackyard, and left for dead there. Two or three hours later, his attacker had decided to stage a shooting accident, and had gone back to the body, only to find the farmer trying to struggle to his feet. A shot had been fired which travelled downwards through the farmer's left arm, knocking him onto his back, and the second shot had been fired from above into his face. The victim had rolled over, and the assailant had again grasped his feet and dragged him, face downwards, into the paddock, finally placing the cap on his head and the gun in his hand.

If, explained Smith to the police, his reconstruction were correct, shotgun pellets ought to be found in the stackyard near the blood stain. A short spell of digging revealed 23 pellets in exactly that area. The farmer's wife and the boy were arrested, and the boy made a full confession, corroborating Smith's findings exactly. He claimed that the wife had suggested the murder, and had attacked the husband with an axe, and that between them they had dragged him from the farmhouse to the stackyard. Some hours later they noticed that the farmer was stirring, and the boy had been handed the gun to finish him off. Afterwards, the wife had placed soil over the bloodstained ground, had buried one cartridge from the gun, and had cleaned and black-leaded the head of the axe.

Despite all this evidence, the wife denied any implication in the killing, and in the absence of any concrete evidence she was found not guilty. The mentally defective boy was found unfit to plead – but at least Professor Smith, with his painstakingly detailed work, had scored a moral victory.

Perhaps the greatest difficulty facing the medico-legal examiner in a doubtful case is in fathoming the mind of the individual involved. Once determined to die, the would-be suicide will on occasion go to the most extraordinary and painful lengths to bring about his own end, often with results which seem quite incredible to the average mind.

A police surgeon from Hull has reported a bizarre case of suicide by multiple means. A man was found hanging, and from the surroundings and the information about him which police investigation uncovered, he had undoubtedly killed himself. The body, however, had a bullet wound in the left side of the face and another in the palm of the left hand, five slashes across the throat, and a gash across the left wrist which had bisected the muscle tendons but not the major blood vessels. The unfortunate man had apparently tried to shoot himself, cut his throat, and slash his wrist, before giving up and hanging himself.

In cases of death from dubious injuries the medical examiner has to answer not only 'how, when and where' questions, but also to what extent the victim could have performed voluntary actions after the injuries were inflicted. The case of Surgey mentioned earlier illustrates the point; he walked over a hundred yards after cutting his throat, despite the massive shock and haemorrhage. If a man is found dead of a bullet wound, say, and a trail of blood leads off for some distance, it is possible that he has been murdered – but far from certain. Even huge damage to the brain may still leave the victim able to function for some time afterwards, as a classic case which occurred in Edinburgh in the 1930s and was reported in the *Police Journal* in 1943 shows.

An elderly professional man, slightly eccentric and living alone in a small private hotel, went out one winter evening and did not return. His disappearance caused no particular alarm, as his habit of walking around at night was well known. The following morning the bell to the street door rang at half past seven, and the maid answered it. On the doorstep stood the man, wearing a hat and heavy overcoat, and carrying his umbrella hooked over one arm. To her consternation, the maid noticed blood on his face and shirt, but he brushed her mildly aside when she moved towards him.

'Don't worry,' he said. 'It's nothing. I'll just go upstairs and have a wash.'

So saying he walked into the hallway, placed his umbrella in the stand, and hung up his hat and coat before going up the stairs to the bathroom. The maid followed him up, and saw him collapse. She called an ambulance and the police, and the old man was taken to the Royal Infirmary, where he died three hours later.

There was no mystery about the cause of death. Under the man's chin was a bullet wound, which tracked upwards through the mouth, through the severely damaged brain, and out through the left-hand side of the top of the skull. The exit wound was about one and a quarter inches in diameter, and suggested a .45 calibre bullet with 'tailwag'; powder stains in the mouth itself seemed to indicate that the man had placed the gun under his chin and pulled the trigger.

The police went back to the hotel and, in freshly fallen snow, traced bloodstained footprints across the road to a small public garden opposite, where on the seat of the shelter, they found a .45 revolver, which was later identified as the property of the dead man. In front of the seat was a large pool of blood, and in the roof of the shelter was a bullet hole, surrounded by fragments of bone and brain tissue; here was where the act had been committed, but the time was more difficult to fix.

The man had left the hotel some time the previous evening and had apparently spent part of the night in the shelter. At six that morning it had begun to snow, and a 165-yard circle of footprints and bloodstains leading from the shelter, out onto the grass, and back to the shelter again, showed that the wound must have been inflicted at around six. Apparently the man had shot himself at about that time, and had sat on the seat with his head hanging forward between his hands, dribbling blood onto the ground. Then he had got up, walked around in a circle, and returned to his starting point once more.

After resting a while longer, he had finally risen to his feet, walked straight across the grass and across the street and rung the doorbell of his hotel.

There he had carried out purposeful acts – hanging up his coat and so on – as well as talking in a lucid manner to the maid, before going upstairs and collapsing. An astounding one and a half hours had elapsed between the suicide bid and his collapse, and he was to live for three more before he finally succumbed to his injuries.

Of course, when sudden death occurs in 'suspicious' circumstances, the police and medical examiner are faced with responsibilities other than that of simply deciding whether or not murder has been committed. On the humane side, the deceased's relatives are entitled to know the precise cause of death, and the insurance companies – where a policy on the dead person's life exists – need to satisfy themselves as to the matter.

The late Professor Cyril J. Polson, in a paper in the *Criminologist* entitled 'Murders that never were' comments:

It is not always wise to accept the claim that death was due to natural causes, regardless of the fact that the circumstances may be consistent with this interpretation; skilled investigation may demonstrate poisoning as the cause . . . The most difficult cases are those of middle-aged and elderly persons who are believed to have died of natural causes and whose bodies contain evidence of natural disease, notably of the coronary arteries, of sufficient severity normally accepted as the cause of death. Routine screening for poisons, notably barbiturates, has shown that, on twelve occasions, the real cause of death was suicide by barbiturate poisoning. The potential for homicidal poisoning exists but so far this routine procedure in my department has not disclosed an instance of it.

Professor Polson recounts several interesting examples of 'murders' that proved to be natural deaths. The captain of a Polish ship en route to Hull radioed for medical help after one of his crew was found lying on deck, surrounded by bloodstains. A doctor was flown out and boarded the vessel, only to find that the man had died; he examined the body as it lay in its cabin and found a stab wound to the left groin, indicating that the man had been the victim of a homicidal attack. Accordingly he radioed the police, and they met the ship when she docked at Hull later in the day.

Initial investigations were highly unsatisfactory; the crew could speak no English and the police had to rely on the ship's captain to act as interprter. One man who had seen the victim immediately before the incident locked himself in his cabin and refused to come out, and when a bloodstain was found on an adjoining cabin door, along with a freshly laundered shirt and trousers, it seemed that the police were dealing with murder.

The body was removed to Hull City Mortuary, where an autopsy was carried out. The police pathologist examined the stab wound and found it to be relatively shallow, for although the femoral vein had been severed the underlying artery was untouched. Probing the wound he found a sliver of glass.

Meanwhile, to one side of the autopsy room a police officer had been going through the pockets of the dead man's clothing; in the left trouser pocket he found several dagger-like shards of glass, with the label from a vodka bottle adhering to them. The mystery was quickly solved. A drinking party had taken place aboard ship, and the dead man had gone for more liquor, picked up the vodka and placed it in his trouser pocket. As he lurched back, slightly drunk, he had slipped on the deck and the bottle had broken, piercing his groin. Because of his intoxication and perhaps shock, he had stumbled around for some time, trying to open the cabin door and thus smearing the handle with blood.

Another apparent stabbing case at first led Yorkshire police to believe that they had a sexual murder on their hands. A young woman was found lying dead in her kitchen, her clothing dishevelled, and with a stab wound in the upper part of her right breast. Medical examination showed that she had not been sexually assaulted, but that her wound had pierced the innominate artery, and she had died of loss of blood.

The investigating officers confirmed that no one had been seen to enter the house that morning, and there was no sign of forced entry. Further enquiry in the house itself showed the cause. At the top of the stairs which led into the kitchen were a chair and a bowl of paste; paper on the wall of the staircase was damp, as if recently applied. The woman had been decorating the staircase, standing on the chair with a pair of trimming scissors in her hand, when she had lost her balance, fallen head-long down the stairs, and impaled herself on the scissors.

Apparently she had plucked them out and thrown them to one side, where they were found. Unfortunately as soon as the scissors were removed from the wound, profuse, fatal bleeding from the severed artery had caused death.

Perhaps the oddest of all methods of self destruction, and one which presents great problems to investigators is also one of the rarest – self-strangulation. As Professor Polson writes:

Throttling raises a strong presumption of murder since accidental throttling is rare and self strangulation by throttling is well nigh impossible. External evidence of throttling is not only abrasion by finger nails but, equally significant and commoner, bruising of the skin of the neck, especially at the front and sides.

Damage to the horns of the delicate hyoid cartilage is also a characteristic mark of murder by throttling; again, however, there are exceptions.

A 66-year old woman was found dead in unusual circumstances. She was lying face downwards on the carpet of her living room, a pair of household steps across her body. Scattered papers and letters in the hearth seemed to indicate a struggle. There was no sign of forced entry, but police learned that she was separated from her husband, who lived in the vicinity, and suspicion fell on him, particularly after the post-mortem. The top of the woman's head bore a scalp wound about an inch long. At the front of her neck slight bruising had occurred, though the neck muscles were unmarked.

However, both horns of the hyoid cartilage were broken at their bases, and fresh bleeding had occurred in the area of the fractures, which were consistent with force being applied to the front of the throat and thrusting the hyoid back against the spine.

Interrogated, the husband proved to have a sound alibi, but he did mention that his wife kept the step ladder, which had been found lying across her body, propped against the wall of the living room. An astute police officer examined the ladder again, measured the distance between the rungs, and checked the measurement against the woman's body. The distance between her head wound and the bruising to her throat proved to be identical with that between the rungs of the ladder. It was concluded that she had had a heart attack and fallen forwards against the ladder, causing the throat damage.

A body found in water has not necessarily drowned, and even if death is proved to be by drowning, did the victim struggle or not ? How long has the body been in the water, and under what conditions ? These are all questions which the forensic medical examiner must answer before the police are able to make a clear start.

A classic example of what can be done by the medico-legal examiner in these directions is the Hopetoun Quarry murder case, which incidentally was the first major investigation conducted by Sydney Smith.

On a Sunday afternoon in 1913 two workmen out for a stroll near Winchburgh, West Lothian, were passing the Hopetoun Quarry, a disused, water-filled crater, when they saw a dark bundle floating near the bank. Curious, they drew the bundle in with a tree branch and discovered to their horror that it was in fact two small bodies tied together with window cord. As they lifted the corpses from the water the cord broke. The police were called, and the bodies were taken to the mortuary at Linlithgow. The local Procurator Fiscal called for a forensic expert, and Sydney Smith was sent for.

Forensic medicine was still in its relatively early state then as an exact science, and the local police doctor felt that there was little point in carrying out an autopsy, as the bodies were badly decomposed, and the features unrecognizable. Such a decision is, as we have seen, a cardinal error still made from time to time today, but the young Smith recognized it as such and insisted on performing a post-mortem.

Firstly, he removed and examined the clothes. Today the clothes of a possible murder victim are examined by the forensic science laboratory technicians, but they are also searched by the medico-legal examiner for they may have much to tell him about the personality, social status, occupation and habits and even state of mind of the deceased. In this particular case however, Smith did not expect too much from the garments, owing to their rotted condition from long immersion. The pathologist had already identified the bodies as those of children, because of their size, and the clothes he removed were typical of the kind worn by small boys of the period – shirts, knicker-bocker trousers, stockings with garters, and boots. Two points struck him instantly; the clothes were of identical make, which seemed to indicate that the children had been brothers or near

60

relatives, and they were of the cheapest possible quality, showing that the victims had been from a poor background. Then Smith found a quite dramatic clue; on the collar of one of the shirts was a faded laundry mark, which when examined with a magnifying glass proved to be that of a poorhouse at Dysart, in Fife.

From a purely medical point of view Smith and his chief, Professor Harvey Littlejohn, were both fascinated by the bodies, because they had undergone an almost complete adipocere change. Normally human fat is semi-fluid, but when a body is immersed for a long period in water or damp earth it gradually converts to a condition known as adipocere, a hardening of the fat into a sort of suet condition, which is permanent when complete. Variable factors affect the time taken for adipocere to set in, but an examination of local conditions can help the pathologist to make a fairly accurate estimate of the time of immersion. In this case Smith calculated that the children had been lying in the water for between eighteen months and two years.

Further examination showed that both were male, and the height and teeth showed their ages to have been respectively six to seven, and four. Both boys' scalps were nearly bare, but small tufts of brown hair on the back showed that they had had close haircuts shortly before death. The elder boy had a small gash on the back of his head, but owing to the adipocerous condition it was impossible to tell whether he had suffered it before or after death. The adipocere became extremely useful again, however, when Smith opened the bodies. The stomachs of each boy had undergone the change, and were completely intact; incredibly, so were their contents. Smith wrote in his autobiography *Mostly Murder*:

In each stomach there were several ounces of thick material, including undigested and easily recognisable vegetable matter – whole green peas, barley, potatoes, turnips, and leeks; in fact the traditional ingredients of Scotch broth. The extensive adipocere formation was responsible for preserving this valuable evidence over such a phenomenally long period. Its importance, of course, was that it helped to fix the time of death. The adipocere itself suggested this was eighteen months to two years ago. Assuming that the vegetables were fresh, the boys' last meal would have been eaten in the late summer or autumn of 1911.

Smith calculated that the meal had been eaten about an hour before death, which suggested that the boys either lived locally, or had not been brought a great distance between the time of the meal and their disposal. With the thoroughness for which he was to become legendary, Smith visited the quarry, which lay a mile east of Winchburgh at the end of a long and winding cart-track.

The chances were that the boys had walked there, not suspecting that they would never walk back. They had walked there with their killer. Then surely they must have known him well. Probably he was a relative. Perhaps even a parent?

And so Smith was able to give the police a sizeable number of facts to go on. Armed with this information, they came to a swift conclusion. Two boys had indeed disappeared suddenly from the neighbourhood in November 1911, although no one had thought much of it at the time as their father, a labourer named Patrick Higgins, had said they were on the way to a relative in Canada. The brothers were aged seven and four, both had brown hair, and both had been in the poor house at Dysart, while their father was in prison for failing to maintain them. Higgins, it appeared, had served as a soldier with distinction in India, and had then returned, taken a job at Winchburgh brickworks and married a local girl. He soon began to drink heavily, however, and had neglected his family; his wife died in 1910, and he had then placed his sons into the care of various local women but had failed to pay for their keep, so that they eventually ended up in the poorhouse.

When he was released from jail he returned to his job and recovered the boys, taking them to live at a shack in the brick-works. One wet and dark night in November a miner named Shields had seen Higgins and the boys 'walking eastwards' – in the direction of the quarry. Later Higgins had returned alone, and had drunk with Shields in a pub. 'The kids are alright now,' he remarked, 'they're on their way to Canada.'

When the police discovered a woman in the area who had taken pity on the boys and given them a meal of Scotch broth one wet November night, and spoke to other people who claimed that Higgins had given contradictory stories to them, their case was closed. Higgins was arrested with ease at his old lodging house and was hanged at Edinburgh in October 1913.

Parts of the adipocerous bodies of the two Higgins boys are preserved in the Forensic Medicine Department at Edinburgh University, and are still used to demonstrate the curious formation to this day.

Adipocere very rarely sets in as extensively as in the Higgins case; sometimes only the fattier portions of the body, the breasts or buttocks, for instance, are preserved in this way while the rest of the body putrefies normally. But adipocere can help the medico-legal examiner put some form of approximate time limit on a body's immersion, whether the condition is almost total or merely fractional.

Drowning is a fairly common cause of sudden death, and the medical examiner needs great diligence to distinguish cases of suicide, accident or murder. Normally if a person who cannot swim falls into deep water he will gasp with shock and inhale liquid into his lungs. Because the body is only slightly heavier than water it sinks but rises again, and the person makes a new effort to clear his lungs, and breathe; usually he breathes in even more water, and the process is repeated again – the classic 'going down for a third time' – until the lungs are waterlogged and the body sinks to the bottom. During the struggle, water is also swallowed.

In a body which has died from drowning, the lungs and air passages are filled with a fine froth, there is water in the stomach, and the lungs 'balloon' with the additional pressure upon them. At the same time the characteristic 'clutching at straws' – or indeed sand or paper or anything floating by – may occur.

If a person is found clutching fragments of clothing or hair which are not his own, the question of homicide must arise, as it must, obviously, where signs of a struggle on dry land are found. But here again, no sudden conclusions should be reached. In one case the floating body of a man was found with his throat cut, the wound having been made before death. There was considerable blood staining on the canal bridge from which he had fallen, and police were able to trace spots of blood back two hundred yards to a deserted house, where they found an open razor on the floor. The first conclusion was that the man had been murdered there, and then dragged to the river, but brief enquiries showed that the man was tenant of the house, and that the prints on the razor were his own – a case of a suicide 'making sure'.

Occasionally, elderly or weakly persons are found dead in baths. Usually they are found to have died of natural causes, such as heart failure or cerebral haemorrhage, or by slipping, knocking themselves unconscious and so drowning. But this particular form of death has been looked upon with great suspicion since the celebrated 'Brides in the bath' case.

In 1915 a man named George Joseph Smith was arrested in England on a 'holding charge' of suspected insurance fraud. In fact the investigating officer, Inspector Arthur Fowler Neil, was convinced that Smith had killed at least three wives, whom he had married under different names – one in Blackpool, one in Highgate, and one in Herne Bay. All had died in the same way, by drowning in their baths, and in every case there were no marks of violence, and local doctors had given the cause of death as heart failure, in one case perhaps due to epilepsy.

Pathologist Bernard Spilsbury was called to re-examine the

*Part of the* Daily Mirror *front page for 2 July 1915, portraying the notorious George Joseph Smith and his women victims (John Frost Historical Newspaper Service).*

bodies, when evidence was produced that they were all connected to Smith, who had claimed insurance money from all their deaths, but for some time neither he nor Inspector Neil could suggest a way in which the women could have been forcibly drowned without signs of violence and without considerable disturbance being heard – all were drowned in boarding houses. One curious circumstance again common to all was that the women were lying with their heads under the water at the sloping end of the bathtub, with their legs sticking out of the other end.

As Spilsbury was later to point out in court, epilepsy causes the body first to contract and then to stretch out, which would have pushed the heads out of the water, while an ordinary faint would have caused water to trickle into the mouth and nostrils, having a reviving effect. A person standing or kneeling while taking a bath might fall forward and be drowned, but then the body would be face downwards. So how had Smith's victims died?

It was Inspector Neil who discovered the answer. Experimenting with a bathing suit-clad policewoman, he asked her to get into a bathtub identical to those used by Smith, and then tried to force her under. Water was splashed everywhere, and strong though he was, Neil could not hold the girl under for more than a few seconds at a time. Then he picked up her legs and pulled; as her head slid under water, she became unconscious immediately – to Neil's horror. It was not until after half an hour's resuscitation that she recovered sufficiently to tell him that the water, rushing up her nose, had shocked her into unconsciousness. Smith was hanged as a result of this evidence.

Drowning is only one of several asphyxial deaths, which briefly are deaths caused by blockage of air to the lungs, thus depriving the brain of vital oxygen.

Suffocation is, of course, frequently caused by fire, where people are trapped in smoke-filled rooms and suffer that perhaps slightly more merciful death before the flames reach them. One of the most dramatic fire deaths in criminal history involved an unknown man, and its importance lies in the fact that the murder might just have succeeded, had the murderer thought his crime through more thoroughly and the police proved slightly more incompetent than they were.

65

November 5 in England is traditionally the day for lighting bonfires and letting off fireworks in memory of Guy Fawkes and the Gunpowder Plot, so two young men walking home to the village of Hardingstone, just south of Northampton, at 2 am on the morning of 6 November 1930, were not surprised to see a bright blaze glowing ahead of them. What did surprise them was to see a fairly smartly dressed man carrying a briefcase hurrying towards them along the lane. He seemed to avert his face as he approached them, but they were able to recognize him later. As he passed he called out: 'Looks like someone's having a bonfire up there'.

Rounding a bend in the lane they saw that the glow was caused by a burning car, a Morris Minor 'baby car' as they were then called. It was completely enveloped, the flames leaping to fifteen feet high, and the heat was intense. One of the young men was the son of the village constable, and ran to fetch his father who called help to douse the flames. Twelve minutes later the flames were out, and the onlookers were horrified to see a blackened human shape lying across the front seats. The village constable did the right thing, and touched nothing; it was an Inspector Lawrence from Northampton who broke the rules which later made the prosecution difficult.

His prime concern was that Hardingstone Lane, in which the car was found, was busy during the day and would, he thought be full of sightseers as soon as the news got out. Instead of cordoning off the area, he moved the still warm remains to the local inn, the *Crown*, leaving the wreckage unguarded for a period of time. Even worse, no notes were taken and no photographs made of the body as it lay where it had apparently died.

Fortunately, the car's registration plates were undamaged, and the vehicle was quickly traced to Alfred Arthur Rouse, who lived in Finchley, North London. Mrs Rouse said that her husband, a commercial traveller, had left home the night before on business. She had not seen him since. The police did not ask her to view the body, which was quite unrecognizable. Meanwhile, Bernard Spilsbury was notified and travelled to Hardingstone to examine the body. It had been hideously damaged, and that in a very short time. The arms and legs were almost burned away, as was the chest wall, and the skull vault was fractured.

66

The lungs showed carbon traces, which meant that the victim had been alive for at least a few seconds after the fire started.

Examination of part of the prostate gland showed that the victim was a man, aged between 21 and 30, and pigment in the lungs indicated to Spilsbury that he had perhaps been a coal miner. He was certain that the skull damage had been caused by the heat, bursting it outwards. But this decision was confused by the discovery of a wooden mallet (which Rouse later admitted belonged to him) by the side of the burned wreckage. On its head were three or four hairs, one of which, admitted Spilsbury, 'had the microscopic characteristics of a human hair . . . That is as far as I think I can safely go.'

In 1947, in the first edition of his *Forensic Medicine*, Dr Keith Simpson contested both Spilsbury's findings as to sex and as to cause of damage to the skull. 'The car was Rouses's,' he wrote, 'but the body was that of a woman, and post-mortem examination showed that she had been murdered by some blunt instrument such as a hammer. Such a weapon was, in fact, found in a ditch nearby.'

Rouse was, of course, the man seen by the two young men in the lane at the murder site. Panicking, he had first gone to Wales, where he was recognized from photographs in the newspapers, and when he returned to London he was arrested. Police discovered a strange history, which also provided a motive. During the First World War he had been wounded in the head by shrapnel, and appeared never to have recovered from his wound. At least from that time on he was a changed man, a compulsive womanizer and fantasist. As a result of his passion for women and his travels as a salesman he had children and several 'wives' all over southern England as well as his own wife in London – at least 80 seductions were traced to him. These had eventually led to money troubles, and he had devised a plan to 'disappear'. He had, he said, contacted a tramp and offered to take him north. He had got the man drunk with whisky, then throttled him and laid him unconscious or dead, he was not sure which, across the seats.

He had then – as police examination confirmed – loosened the petrol union joint, removed the carburettor, leaked petrol on to the road, and ignited it. Rouse was tried and executed.

There was a strange sequel to this sensational case two years later. A man with the appropriate name of Furnace, who had a small building firm in Hawley Crescent, Camden Town, also got into financial trouble, and remembered the Rouse case. Rouse, he decided – naively – had only made the mistake of being seen leaving the scene of the crime. Furnace decided to imitate him, but to do the deed on covered premises. In January 1933, he lured a young acquaintance named Spatchett into his workshop and shot him in the back. He then waited until after midnight, stripped the body of identification and the considerable sum of money which Spatchett had been carrying, and poured oil and paint over the body and the furniture. He had left a note in his apartment to the effect that he was going to commit suicide, and now he set fire to the building, ducked unseen through the back streets, and reached Southend, where he took lodgings and posed as an invalid.

The fire devastated the building and blistered the body beyond ordinary recognition. Furnace's note was found and the police reported the death as suicide by the builder. Unfortunately the body had been sitting on a stool, a circumstance which the North London coroner, Bentley Purchase, thought odd. He visited the premises himself, examined the body and found a hole in the back which proved to be a bullet wound. Furnace, like other fire killers, had either forgotten or did not know that teeth are virtually indestructible, and those of the corpse were proved to belong to a much younger man. Intensive investigation showed the body to be that of Spatchett, and after a hue and cry which lasted for a fortnight Furnace was traced and arrested. He, however, unlike his mentor Rouse, escaped the gallows by managing to smuggle a bottle of drugs into the police station with him, and this time really committing suicide.

The final form of asphyxial death most likely to concern the forensic pathologist is hanging, and the distinction between this and strangulation is very important for a number of reasons, the main one being the differentiation between a genuine, suicidal hanging and homicide which has been made to look like suicide.

Where suicidal hanging is concerned death is due to either rupture or obstruction of blood vessels in the brain due to pressure on the vessels of the neck, or obstruction of the wind-pipe, or both. The rope or ligature used leaves a deep bruise on the flesh at the point of pressure, so that the examiner can tell, even if the rope has been removed, whether or not for instance the delicate bones of the hyoid cartilage have been broken by the rope or by manual strangulation. As bruising is caused by the breaking of the tiny capillary blood vessels, a rope put around the neck after death would not normally show much of a mark when removed at all. Several of these factors were involved in the controversial Thorne case.

Norman Thorne was a lower middle class poultry farmer who occasionally attended the Wesleyan chapel at Crowborough, Sussex, where he had grown up. In 1922 he had entered the poultry business, and struggled for two years to make his piece of land with ramshackle outbuildings in the hamlet of Blackness pay its way. In 1924, when he was just as old as the century, he had become entangled with a neurotic girl named Elsie Cameron, who wanted to marry him, but who meanwhile was willing to sleep with him occasionally in the converted brooding shed on his allotment. She lived some distance away, however, and during one of her absences Thorne got to know a rather more attractive girl nearby, Elizabeth Coldicott.

Elsie Cameron heard of the new involvement, and stormed to Thorne's home, claiming to be pregnant – which she was not – and demanding instant marriage. She arrived on 5 December, and was never seen alive again.

Five days later her father telegraphed to find out what had become of her, and Thorne replied that he did not know; he had been expecting her on the morning of the sixth. Crowborough police were called by Mr Cameron, and found the dull but respectable Thorne anxious to be helpful; he appeared genuinely worried about the fate of his fiancée, and called at Crowborough police station during the next few days with helpful suggestions and constant requests for news. When the press heard of the mystery Thorne happily told them about his 'forthcoming marriage' to Elsie, and posed for them in his chicken run; in a curious act of bravado he stood for one photograph in exactly the spot where her body was later found. Two men who vaguely knew Elsie claimed to have seen her turning in to the lane leading to Thorne's farm on the night in question, but the Crowborough police appear to have dismissed the notion. But about a month later, when a woman neighbour who had been away and had not heard of the mystery returned, she repeated the story and Scotland Yard were informed. Thorne himself repeated his earlier story at Crowborough to the Yard men, unaware that digging had already begun at his farm. The following day Elsie's dressing case was discovered, and Thorne was detained. With a sigh, he made his final statement. Elsie had arrived, he said, and had sworn that she would stay until he married her. He had told her that he needed time to think, and had gone out to meet his other girl, Elizabeth Coldicott. When he returned late in the evening, he had found Elsie swinging by a noose from the hut's main beam. Thorne claimed that he had panicked – the usual line taken by such killers – had cut off Elsie's head and legs, and had buried these and the trunk in his hen-run.

The following day Elsie's butchered remains were dug up and taken to the local mortuary, where Spilsbury examined them. There were bruises on the head, face, elbow, legs and feet 'which together' he said, 'were amply sufficient to account for death from shock, death which must have occurred very shortly after those injuries were inflicted'. Of course, because of the suggestion of hanging, he examined the neck for bruises, not only externally, but in the tissues under the skin. Cutting across what he claimed were the 'natural' creases of the neck, he found no evidence of haemorrhage which might be consistent with hanging. On January 26, the remains were taken for official burial in Willesden graveyard. But the matter was not allowed to rest there; Spilsbury was to appear for the prosecution, under Sir Henry Curtis-Bennett. Sir James Cassels, appearing for the defence, decided to get a second opinion, in the person of Dr Robert Bronte, then pathologist at Harrow Hospital and a former Crown Analyst to the Irish Government, prior to the establishment of the Irish Free State in 1922.

A second post-mortem was ordered, and in late February, nearly three months after Elsie had died, her body was disinterred for a second examination by Bronte, at which Spilsbury was present.

The battle of the two men at the subsequent trial was one which was to have far-reaching repercussions. It was the first time that Spilsbury had ever been seriously challenged on his own ground – particularly on the subject of bruising, on which he had become a specialist even at that stage of his career. Spilsbury maintained that two bruises in particular – on Elsie's head and cheek – had probably been the fatal ones, causing crushing of tissues. Bronte argued that such blows would have caused tearing of the skin and chipping of the cheekbone, which they had not done. but nevertheless had to admit that his post-mortem had taken place when the body was in an advanced state of decomposition.

The defence then suggested that the body had been subjected to an attempted hanging by the girl herself, that she had been found suspended but still alive by Thorne, but had died soon afterwards from shock and congestion to the brain.

Spilsbury immediately claimed that he had seen no sign at all of congestion to the brain during the first post-mortem, and said that the action of water on the body in the intervening period before the second autopsy had destroyed the tissues so that no extravesion – bruising – could be seen. However, he pointed out, hanging or attempted hanging would have left immediate marks on the neck, and there were none to be seen. There were no marks except 'natural creases', and he had examined these thoroughly but not, he admitted, microscopically at the first post-mortem because it was unnecessary at that time.

Dr Bronte described the marks he had found as 'grooves' and claimed that bruising had been visible on them. He had taken slides of them and had passed sections of the bruised areas to Spilsbury, who had made his own slides from them. Spilsbury testified that on neither his slides, nor those of Bronte, were any signs of bruising to be observed.

Spilsbury made one final, telling point, after the testimony of Thorne. Thorne claimed that when he found Elsie hanging, 'her eyes were open, but screwed up'.

On the last morning of the trial Spilsbury refuted this. 'Assuming unconsciousness had intervened, if not death, the eyes would have been in the condition of paralysis. That is to say, the eyes would not have been completely closed, or com-

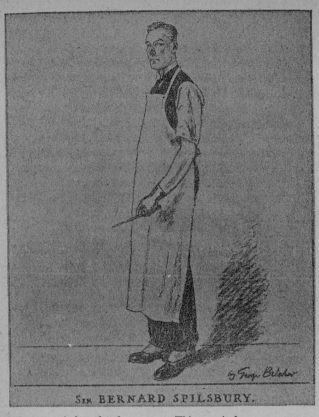

SIR BERNARD SPILSBURY.

*When arsenic has closed your eyes, This certain hope your corpse may rest in:– Sir B. will kindly analyse The contents of your large intestine. A cartoon by George Belcher which appeared, with this verse beneath it, in the pages of* Punch (*John Topham Picture Library*).

pletely open; a half-open condition, with flexive lids; certainly no puckering.'

The judge, in his summing up, said that Spilsbury's was 'undoubtedly the very best opinion that can be obtained' and that although perhaps there might have been some slight bruising on the girl's neck, it could hardly have been caused by hanging.

The jury agreed, and Thorne was sentenced to death. There now followed a huge outcry in the press claiming that Thorne had been unfairly tried; among the leaders were Arthur Conan Doyle – who claimed that there was a 'faint doubt existing' – and the editor of the *Law Journal*. But the appeal was unsuccessful, and Thorne was executed.

The oddities of accident in suspicious deaths and attempted suicides are perhaps best illustrated by the allegedly true story beloved by lecturers in forensic medicine for its nice portrayal of the part which can be played by coincidence.

A would-be suicide had spent some time considering what course of self destruction he would take, and eventually hit upon what appeared to be a fool-proof plan. He selected the stout branch of a tree which jutted from a sheer cliff face overlooking the sea as a good place from which to hang himself. In order to prevent any pain, however, he swallowed a large dose of opium, and in case the drop was not sufficient and he was in danger of dying by slow strangulation, loaded a pistol to carry with him.

At the site he tied a rope around the branch with the other end around his neck and jumped, the pistol held over his head. Unfortunately the pistol went off, partly severing the rope, and the jerk of his body parted the last few strands. He fell fifty feet into the sea below, swallowed salt water and vomited up the opium before swimming ashore, vowing never to try to kill himself again.

# Chapter Four
# These vile guns

With windy nitre and quick sulphur fraught
And ramm'd with bullet round, ordain'd to kill.

Edmund Spenser, *Faerie Queen*, Book 1

Around the year 1515, a new invention reached the shores of England from the Continent. It was said to have originated in the Italian town of Pistoia, whence it derived its name, but it first arrived in London from Germany. It was the wheel-lock pistol, and it was to start the first truly modern trend in crime – robbery and murder with a firearm.

King Henry VIII, then a carefree sportsman a full decade away from the matrimonial problems which were to bring him into conflict with the Pope, at first looked upon the import with interest. He was already a relatively skilled marksman with the arquebus, the clumsy forerunner of the musket and carbine, and he took up the new weapon with enthusiasm. But within a few years a minor crime wave on the highways leading into London and other major cities had caused him to have second thoughts. 'Evil disposed persons,' he wrote, 'have done detestable murders with little short guns.'

Though the wheel-lock was neither little nor short by modern standards, it was portable, and for the next two centuries the pistol – whether wheel-lock, snaphaunce or flint-lock – featured in hundreds of crimes, many of them unsolved. It was not until another crime wave – that which followed the introduction of Prohibition in the 1920s and plunged the United States into an era of firearm-backed lawlessness – that criminologists were forced to look more closely at guns and their properties. The result was the science which has the specific title of forensic ballistics. Nigel Morland writes in his *Scientific Criminology*,

Forensic ballistics is not regarded as a wholly acceptable definition of what is actually firearms identification, but the Oxford English Dictionary accepts ballistics as the science of projectiles in flight, hence the misnomer; forensic is its own qualification, and the definition is to be preferred to elaborations which may say more, but mean no more than the handier description. Experts in this field of work usually refer to each other as 'firearms examiners'.

Firearms examiners are principally concerned with whether or not a particular bullet was fired from a particular gun, the range at which the shot was fired, and the approximate time when a weapon was last fired; they also combine with the forensic pathologist to study the cause, nature and effect of bullet wounds. Taking these factors into consideration we can say that the first known case of 'forensic ballistics' being used in court took place as far back as 1784.

In that year the body of a man named Edward Culshaw was found with a gunshot wound to the head, and an acquaintance of his, John Toms, was arrested on suspicion. Toms was the owner of a muzzle-loading flintlock pistol. To load such a weapon, gunpowder was first poured down the barrel and a paper wad was tamped down on top of it with a ramrod. Next the ball was pushed into the barrel, and a further paper wad was jammed in to stop the ball falling out. Frequently, the heavy ball would carry pieces of the second wad into the wound with it, and this had occurred in the case of Culshaw; probing of the wound revealed a piece of paper which had been folded over several times to increase its thickness.

When this was cleaned and unfolded, it proved to be a strip of paper torn from a broadsheet, or early newspaper. In John Toms' pocket was the rest of the broadsheet, its frayed edge matching that of the paper wad perfectly. This early piece of 'scientific' evidence sent Toms to the gallows.

The next recorded case is in the memoirs of Henry Goddard, one of the last of the famous Bow Street Runners who immediately preceded the Metropolitan Police as guardians of London's law. In 1835, Goddard was called to the scene of a shooting and examined the leaden ball extracted from the dead man by a surgeon. Like almost all bullets in use with the firearms of that time it was home-made, cast in a mould, and it bore a curious ridge. Goddard had several suspects in mind and he visited them all in turn, asking to see their bullet moulds. In one of these an indentation exactly matched the ridge on the murder bullet, and Goddard was able to secure a conviction. This case foreshadowed the standard procedures of the twentieth-century firearms examiners.

In 1860, yet another murder case concerning a wad created a stir. A police constable was shot and killed in Lincoln, England, and investigators found a wad lying near the body. It was singed and smelled of sulphur, but when unfolded it proved to be a piece of newspaper bearing the title and date of publication: *The Times*, 27 March 1854. At a suspect's home a double-barrelled pistol was recovered with one barrel discharged. When the other barrel was unloaded it was found that the ball had also been tamped with a newspaper wad. The editor of *The Times* was able to show the judge at Lincoln Assizes that the wad from the unfired barrel came from the same edition of his paper as that found by the body. As a result, the pistol's owner, one Richardson, was convicted and hanged.

All these early cases, of course, were somewhat fortuitous, relying on the examiners' powers of deduction rather than on any scientific basis. But already such pioneer criminologists as the Austrian, Hans Gross, were pondering the possibility of identifying bullets and powder. Gross, an examining judge who later compiled the classic *Criminal Investigation*, relates how a family relic turned his thoughts in the direction of forensic ballistics. His grandfather, while serving in the Austrian army in 1799, had been shot in the head by a soldier in Napoleon's forces. The ball lodged behind his eye, and remained there until his death in 1845, two years before Gross's birth. The bullet was removed from the body and kept as a memento; when Gross saw it years later he noticed immediately that traces of powder adhered to it. Could such an occurrence ever have significance in the course of a criminal investigation? Gross felt so, but the 'how' of such matters was not to be perfected for another half century.

In the United States in particular, the nineteenth century brought problems so far as gun killings were concerned. Thousands of American citizens took advantage of their right to bear arms, embodied in the Constitution, following the opening of the West and the great Civil War. On the frontier the slightest disputes were 'settled' with Samuel Colt's cap-and-ball revolvers, and numerous accidents occurred when miners and cowboys discharged their weapons through sheer high spirits. Such wildly erractic firearms as the Adams 'pepperbox' pistol were in great demand; in effect the Adams consisted of nine barrels welded together which were meant to rotate one at a time under the hammer. More often than not, however, all nine barrels discharged at once. scattering lethal balls in all directions. As Mark Twain remarked after handling a pepperbox in the Nevada minefields, it was 'so infernal *comprehensive*'.

Under such circumstances, gun murders were almost impossible to prove, and only eyewitness evidence, often doubtful in the extreme, could be used to convict killers. Attempts were made, however, to introduce 'scientific' evidence into court.

In 1879 a man named Moughton was charged with killing an adversary with two shots from his revolver. Moughton claimed that, though he owned a pistol, he had not fired it for over a year and the judge, apparently progressive in his outlook, asked a gunsmith to examine the disputed weapon. The gunsmith squinted down the barrel and pronounced that as it was 'mildewed' and 'full of rust' it could not have been fired for at least 18 months. Primitive evidence, again, by contemporary standards, but it secured the defendant's acquittal.

It was the widespread introduction of rifling in the nineteenth century, along with the development of the brass cartridge, which brought about the first real possibility of firearm identification. Rifling – the cutting of spiral grooves into the interior of a gun-barrel in order to spin the projectile and keep it travelling on a straight line – was far from new, but a serious objection to rifling lay in the difficulty of ramming a ball down the barrel of a muzzle-loader. This problem was resolved to a certain extent when the first breech-loading guns were introduced towards the end of the eighteenth century.

Colt's revolvers, first patented in 1835, were rifled, though his early models, such as the Dragoon, the Walker and the Navy Colts, were 'cap-and-ball' weapons. It was only after 1866, with the introduction of the brass cartridge, that the Colt factory were able to produce their classic 'Frontier' pistol, the familiar 'Gun That Won The West' which was also ironically nicknamed the 'Peacemaker'. More or less simultaneously the

Winchester Rifle Company introduced their repeating carbine, which also used brass cartridges, and within a few months rivals of Colt and Winchester, both in the United States and in Europe, were mass-producing weapons along similar lines.

The effect of rifling on the elongated bullet fired from a brass cartridge was vital to the development of forensic ballistics, though no one noticed the fact for some time. Manufacturers differed in the number of grooves they cut into their barrels; some used four, others used up to seven, and the width of the grooves and the 'lands' – the smooth surfaces between them – also differed. The number of windings, the angle of the grooves, and the direction of twist – which determined whether the bullet spun to right or left – were equally varied. Because the cartridge fitted tightly into the barrel, the grooves and lands marked it as it left the gun, and these marks were to prove to be distinctive.

As far as is known, the first criminologist to make practical use of these facts was Professor Alexandre Lacassagne, France's leading nineteenth-century forensic pathologist, who founded the medico-legal department at Lyons University. In the spring of 1889, during an autopsy on a gunshot victim, Lacassagne removed a bullet from the corpse and examined it carefully. Seven longitudinal grooves were noticeable on its surface, and the Professor deduced that these had been made by rifling in the barrel of the murder weapon. Shown a number of pistols owned by suspects, Lacassagne found only one with seven grooves, and on the basis of this discovery the owner was convicted. Indubitably the Professor was working on the right lines, but with hindsight the court's decision was one that causes deep unease among modern firearms examiners. It is quite possible that different arms manufacturers could have made several different types of seven-grooved revolvers and that the suspect's gun was not, in this case, the murder weapon.

Nine years later Paul Jeserich, a forensic chemist at the University of Berlin, was involved in a similar case, in the small German town of Neuruppin. He was given a suspect revolver and a bullet taken from the body of a murdered man. The idea was that Jeserich, who had little or no experience in the ballistics field, should conduct chemical tests on the weapon and missile. But when Jeserich fired a test bullet from the gun and compared it with the murder bullet, he noticed what appeared to be identical abnormalities on the two surfaces. He took microphotographs of the two missiles and comparison of the markings showed them to be identical; largely because of this testimony a conviction was secured, though the significance of his work appears to have passed Jeserich by; he returned to his field of forensic chemistry and took little further interest in the subject of ballistics.

Back in the United States, however, more and more interest was being shown in the problem, to such an extent that small-town gunsmiths and far less qualified individuals were setting themselves up as 'ballistics' experts. Out of the resulting babble one sane voice spoke but went largely unheard; it was that of Dr A. Llewellyn Hall, who in 1900 published *The Missile and the Weapon*. The book outlined the problems of firearm identification and foreshadowed their solution with great accuracy, and it caught the attention of the great jurist and author Oliver Wendell Holmes.

Two years after the publication of Dr Llewellyn Hall's monograph, Holmes was the presiding judge in a Massachusetts court when a man named Best went on trial for murder. Best had allegedly killed his victim with a revolver and Holmes, remembering what he had read in the New York doctor's booklet, called in a gunsmith to examine the evidence. The gunsmith fired a test shot from Best's gun into a box containing wadded cotton wool – a technique still used today – and then, uusing a magnifying glass and a microscope, pointed out the points of correspondence between the two bullets to the jury. Holmes was most impressed, stating in his summing up: 'I see no other way in which the jury could have learned so intelligently how a gun barrel would have marked a lead bullet fired through it.'

In Europe the budding science of forensic ballistics was still in the hands, not of gunsmiths, but of forensic pathologists; indeed right until the middle of the present century criminologists were to argue that this was how it should be, so closely linked was the bullet to the wound which it inflicted. In 1905 Richard Keckel, head of the Institute of Forensic Medicine at Leipzig University, proposed an interesting but ultimately abortive plan for taking impressions of bullets by rolling them across sheets composed of wax and zinc white, in order to obtain negatives of the missiles' complete surfaces.

Much more important was a development announced by the Frenchman Balthazard, also a practitioner of forensic medicine, in 1913. He had noticed that not only the bullet but the brass cartridge case was marked when a gun fired. The firing pin naturally left an indentation on the detonator cap of the cartridge case, but also the breech block, against which the case was slammed with tremendous force as the charge exploded, impressing itself on the relatively soft metal. These marks appeared to differ from weapon to weapon, commented Balthazard, but much more data needed to be accumulated before accurate deductions could be made.

Ironically, all the data anyone could wish for in the field of ballistics was to be made available in the following four years, as the Great War broke upon the world. Millions of men died by the bullet, yet such were the pressures of society on both sides of the Atlantic and both sides of the trenches that only a tiny handful of men pushed ahead with the pioneering work. One of the greatest of these was Charles E. Waite, whose passion for gathering data in the sphere of forensic ballistics was to equal that shown by Alphonse Bertillon a half century before in the field of anthropometry (see Chapter 6).

In July 1917, when Waite became involved in criminal ballistics for the first time, he was a middle-aged man working as an assistant investigator in the office of the New York State Prosecutor.

A two-year-old murder case had so vexed public opinion that it was drawn to the attention of Governor Whitman of New York, and Whitman set up a special commission to investigate the case anew. The commission was headed by a lawyer from Syracuse named George H. Bond, and he chose the plodding but reliable Waite to be his personal assistant.

The case had begun sometime during the early hours of a dark March night in 1915. A seventy-year-old farmer named Charles B. Phelps had been found dying of a gunshot wound on his farm at West Shelby, in Orleans County, New York.

Nearby lay the body of his housekeeper, Margaret Wolcott; like Phelps she had been shot with a .22 calibre weapon. When Phelps died without regaining consciousness, Sheriff Chester Bartlet went to the farm and arrested a hired hand, Charlie Stielow, who had first reported the killings.

Stielow was a half-witted German immigrant who spoke little English. At first he denied the crime, but when police found a .22 pistol in his quarters he first blustered that he had hidden the weapon out of fear, and then broke down and made a confession admitting his guilt. When he appeared in court, however, he retracted the confession, claiming that he had been promised his freedom if he admitted to the crime.

Appearing for the prosecution was one of the many charlatan 'experts' on ballistics who had appeared in American legal circles during the past two decades or so; the self-styled 'Doctor' Albert Hamilton.

Hamilton made great play of examining Stielow's pistol barrel and the bullets taken from the bodies. He alleged that a scratch in the muzzle of Stielow's .22 corresponded with a mark on the bullets – though neither the judge nor the defence lawyer could discern it. Indeed the judge had grave doubts about the whole case; for one thing no trace of money, said to have been stolen from Phelps' homestead, was found in Stielow's quarters, and his family had had to bring grave hardship upon themselves by selling their only cow for his defence. Nevertheless he was found guilty and on 23 July 1915 he was sent to Sing Sing to await execution.

Several attempts were made to gain a re-trial and though none of these was successful, Stielow's defence attorneys managed to gain a stay of execution in July 1916, after their client had actually been strapped to the electric chair. Then two tramps named King and O'Connell confessed to killing Phelps, and as a result of this turn of events Governor Whitman stepped in.

Bond and his assistant Waite went over the entire evidence again. After questioning the police, Stielow, and the two vagrants King and O'Connell, they came to the private conclusion that the latter were the real culprits, but they were still faced with the 'evidence' put forward by Hamilton. Then Waite remembered a friend of his on the New York City homicide squad, a Captain Jones, who had made a lifelong study of handguns. Captain Jones examined Stielow's revolver and found the barrel badly corroded. In his opinion it could not have been fired for about four or five years – long before the murder was committed.

Despite the danger presented by the rusty barrel, Jones test-fired two bullets from the revolver; one into a barrel of water, the other into a box of cotton waste. The difference between the test bullets and those taken from the bodies was immediately apparent. The latter were clean and lightly marked, while the former were ingrained with rust from Stielow's pistol.

Charles Waite was now convinced of Stielow's innocence, but he needed absolute proof. He sent both sets of bullets to a laboratory of applied optics and microscopy at Rochester. There an expert showed that though both bullets had five lands and grooves, those on the murder bullets were twice as broad as those on the test bullets. This evidence was incontestable, and Governor Whitman gave Charlie Stielow a free pardon.

Waite was enormously elated by his success, but he realized, as the Frenchman Balthazard had done before the war, that a great deal of data had to be collected before positive identification of weapons could be achieved. In 1920, after serving two years with the Army, he set out to collate this data.

For two years he travelled around every major gun manufacturer in the United States – Colt, Remington, Smith & Wesson, Winchester and the rest – asking for the specifications of every weapon they had ever made – the grooves, lands, direction of twist, and calibre. Unfortunately, as he discovered when his American tour was at an end, over two-thirds of the firearms used in crime in the country at that period were of European manufacture, brought back by returning servicemen. Despite the setback of a weak heart, Waite was undaunted. At the end of 1922 he sailed for Europe and repeated his researches there. While in Austria, he made a discovery which was to be vital to the perfection of forensic ballistics as an exact science. Examining the cutting tools which reamed out the grooves in gun barrels, he found that each one left its individual mark; it had to be sharpened regularly, and as its edge wore away the tiny 'teeth' which made up the edge altered minutely. This meant that the marks made by the barrel's grooves and lands – 'striations' as they came to be called – ought to be truly individual.

Waite returned to the United States at the end of 1922, and immediately began to assemble a team of experts who would help to bear out his theories. His researches had stirred up interest in the world of criminology and he was fortunate to attract two men who were to become as dedicated as Waite himself; in fact each was to add an instrument to the world's forensic science laboratories.

John H. Fischer was a physicist who worked with the Bureau of Standards and had always had an interest in firearms. When he heard Waite expound his theory of 'individual striations' he realized that an ability to inspect the interior of gun barrels would be a major asset. Fischer had worked with the cystoscope, a medical instrument used to insert fine tubes carrying lamps into the bladder and kidneys to enable doctors to examine them without resorting to an operation. Adapted, the cystoscope would be ideal. After a period of experiment, Fischer came up with the helixometer. Like its forerunner it consisted of a long hollow probe fitted with a lamp which could be inserted into the muzzle of a gun; it also had a magnifying apparatus at its tail-end which permitted examination of the interior on a large scale.

Waite's second disciple was a distinguished chemist and microphotographer named Philip O. Gravelle. His contribution to forensic ballistics was to be if anything more important than those made by Fischer and Waite himself: he invented the comparison microscope. In essence this comprised two microscope objectives joined by one viewing lens; two bullets could be placed end to end under this instrument and, magnified, could be easily compared for correspondence or dissimilarities.

With these two instruments, firearms examiners can now determine the number, width and direction of rifling grooves and the 'pitch' of rifling – the angle of the spiral. They do this by microscopic examination of the bullet found at the scene of the crime and they can achieve considerable accuracy today even though the bullet has been damaged on impact. If they have access to the alleged weapon used in the crime they can then examine the interior of the barrel, using the helixometer, before test firing the gun to produce a bullet for comparison under the microscope. Matters are greatly helped if the criminal has been careless enough to leave an empty cartridge case behind, for the marks left on this can be as informative as those on the actual projected bullet.

When a firearm is discharged (except those using rim-fire ammunition) the firing pin falls onto a soft metal cap at the rear end of the cartridge which is filled with a detonating compound and which sends a flash through a tiny hole into the main body of the powder-filled case, exploding it and forcing the bullet out. The force is tremendous – in a hand gun it can be as much as four or five tons to the square inch – and the cartridge is both blown back against the breech block and expanded against the walls of the firing chamber. Any tooling marks on the interior surface of the gun are thus imprinted onto the cartridge metal.

The work of Waite and, in particular, Gravelle, convinced the American authorities that a new and official approach should be made to the problem of crime involving firearms, for by this time Prohibition was spawning those gangs of mobsters whose shoot-outs were to make the activities of Western outlaws of the previous century pallid by comparison. The result was the New York based Bureau of Forensic Ballistics, the first organization of its kind in the world. Founded shortly before New Year 1923, the Bureau was to ensure America's leading place in the field for the next half century.

But the man who was to make this so was a comparative late-comer. Colonel Calvin Goddard, a native of Baltimore, was a doctor by training and until joining the army had been a promising heart surgeon. Serving in France, his abiding interest in firearms, as intense as that of Fischer's, caused him to transfer from the Medical Corps to Ordnance.

In 1920 he had returned to the United States, civilian life, and medicine, but his taste for guns was still overwhelming. When he met Waite in 1925 and heard his ideas, Goddard immediately agreed to join the three-year-old Bureau. He threw himself so enthusiastically into his work that, when Waite died just over a year later, Goddard was already his natural successor as head of the Bureau of Forensic Ballistics.

Those criminologists in Europe who noted Goddard's appointment felt that it was natural enough that a medical man should turn gun expert, for whenever forensic evidence was required in cases of firearms' deaths they were almost automatically referred to the nearest forensic pathologist – a trend set by Professor Lacassagne years earlier. A case involving Bernard Spilsbury, for instance, had caused a minor sensation in the last year of the war.

One January night in 1918 a shot rang out in the barracks of the Canadian Corps, stationed at Warminster, Wiltshire. A Corporal Dunkin was found sprawled on his bed, with the bedclothes drawn up to his chin and his arms dangling on either side of the narrow cot. On the floor lay a .303 Lee-Enfield rifle with the breech open. By it was an ejected shell. The bullet had hit Dunkin in the left temple and exited just behind his right ear, passing through his pillow, kitbag, and the hut wall before embedding itself in the ground outside. The local police were inclined to believe that the corporal had committed suicide, but nevertheless Spilsbury was called in to perform a post-mortem.

When he saw the body *in situ*, Spilsbury was struck by the almost abnormal shortness of the dead man's arms in relation to his height of 5 feet 7½ inches. From markings around the entrance wound he estimated that the gun muzzle had been at a distance of at least five inches from Dunkin's temple at the time the shot was fired, and he was able to show that it was manifestly impossible for him to have reached the trigger of the gun from his supine position, much less worked the bolt. As a result the police conducted a thorough investigation and finally arrested a private named Asser, who had killed Dunkin because of a grudge.

But the Dunkin affair created the newspaper stir it did simply because it was a rarity; Britain, like most of the European mainland, had little in the way of gun crime, and in any case forensic medicine had been involved more than forensic ballistics. Nevertheless it was an up-and-coming medico-legal man, the brilliant and volatile Professor Sydney Smith, who brought European legal ballistics into line with its American counterpart.

A year before the Dunkin case, Smith was appointed medico-legal adviser to the Egyptian Government, which was then, of course, British. After the war the native Egyptians began to agitate for independence, and in the first five years of Smith's incumbency at the Government forensic laboratory – which he more or less single-handedly set up – there were 30 murders or attempted murders of officials by shooting, five by means of home-made bombs, and innumerable firearm incidents involving the Egyptians themselves. In none of the political cases did the police manage to make an arrest, and so Smith took it upon himself to collect the bullets and where possible the weapons used in the killings and to build up a file, doing on a small scale what Waite was doing.

On two occasions he embarrassed the Government. In the first instance he discovered that several Egyptians killed in a riot had been shot with square-tipped bullets of a kind issued to the Ghaffirs, an irregular force attached to the police. Some time later he found that rioters in Alexandria had been killed by British Army type .303 bullets, which were of a peculiar design at the time. His reports were suppressed, but he carried on collecting the information. When, in mid-1924, he noticed a paragraph in a science journal which dealt with Gravelle's comparison microscope, he built one himself. It was fortunate timing, for a few months later he was to be involved in his first major ballistics case.

On 19 November 1924, Sir Lee Stack, the British Sirdar (Commander-in-Chief) in Egypt, was being driven back from lunch at the Cairo War Office with his aide-de-camp when his car was riddled with bullets. Stack, his aide, Captain Patrick Campbell, and the driver were all hit, and the Sirdar died of his wounds the following day. At the scene of the crime Smith found nine cartridge shells, and later removed six bullets from the wounded men. All nine shells were .32 calibre, though three different guns had been used: one of them, judging by ejector marks, was a Colt automatic. The bullets were more informative.

Five of them had had crosses filed into their noses to make them into 'dum dum' projectiles – designed to cause massive wounding. From the grooves and their direction of twist it was possible to tell that the bullets had been fired from a Colt automatic, a Mauser automatic, and either a Browning or a Sûreté automatic – Smith's experience was limited at this time and he could not be sure of the third weapon.

Using their widespread network of informers, the Cairo police meanwhile gained the names of four suspects: two brothers named Enayat, a lawyer named Shafik Mansur and another man named Mahmoud Rashid. There was no firm evidence against them, but the police tricked the brothers Enayat into fleeing, then arrested them and discovered four hidden pistols in their luggage. Two of the pistols were eliminated, being of .25 calibre. The other two, a Colt and a Sûreté, were .32 calibre and Smith was able to identify them as being the murder weapons. In fact the Colt had a distinctive flaw which told him that it had been used in several previous unsolved murders. At Rashid's home further evidence came to light; various tools and a sprinkling of nickel, copper and lead filings showed Smith that the dum dum bullets had been made there; to clinch matters, police found a hidden compartment in a doorway, into which the weapons fitted neatly, scratch marks on the woodwork showing where the foresights of the pistols had rested.

Smith was naturally elated by his first major success in the ballistics field, and contributed a paper on the case to the *British Medical Journal*. The same year he devoted a section of his *Textbook of Forensic Medicine* to the problems of forensic ballistics, and it was through these writings that the attention of the European criminological world was finally focused on the new branch of their science.

In the United States another *cause célèbre* was to set the final seal of official approval on Colonel Goddard's Bureau of Forensic Ballistics. This was the Sacco and Vanzetti case, which for the best part of seven years occupied the front pages of the world's newspapers, as left-wing intellectuals clamoured for 'justice' and in so doing made political martyrs of the two principals.

The case began on Christmas Eve 1919, when a car load of

'foreign looking' men attempted to hi-jack the payroll of a small factory in Bridgewater, Massachusetts. The men exchanged fire with guards, and left behind a spent shotgun cartridge, though no one was hurt.

On 15 April 1920, a similar hi-jacking was more successful. Two men leapt from a car outside a shoe factory at South Braintree, not far from Bridgewater, shot down two employees, Parmenter and Berardelli, snatched $16,000 and drove off; eye witnesses claimed that three other men were in the get-away car. Berardelli died instantly, with four .32 calibre bullets in his chest; by his body four ejected .32 automatic cartridges were found. Parmenter was critically wounded and died some hours later, again of a .32 bullet wound. The bullets and the empty shells were found to have been manufactured by the firms of Winchester, Peters, and Remington.

Some time later two men were arrested on a Bridgewater street car. They were 29-year-old Nicola Sacco, a shoemaker, and 32-year-old Bartolomeo Vanzetti, a fishmonger. Both were self-confessed anarchists, and at the time of their arrest Sacco was armed with a .32 calibre Colt automatic, plus twenty-three .32 calibre bullets variously manufactured by Winchester, Remington, and Peters.

Vanzetti carried a .38 calibre Harrington-Richardson revolver; in addition he had four shotgun shells in his pocket similar to the one found empty at the site of the Bridgewater robbery.

At the time the United States had suffered a spate of 'anarchist' outrages, with home-made bombs being thrown at the houses of such men as John D. Rockefeller, and fire bombs being posted to prominent Senators and government officials. The immediate cause appeared to be the unrest in industrial areas of the east coast, caused by primitive conditions of employment among immigrant workers. The arrest of the two Italians, who had immigrated to the United States in 1908, gave the authorities a scapegoat and the workers a rallying cry.

It was under these emotional conditions that Sacco and Vanzetti were brought to trial for the first time. Vanzetti was charged with being implicated in the Bridgewater attack, though Sacco had a firm alibi for that date. In the South Braintree case,

VOL. LXVIII. NO. 24,582—DAILY.          NEW YORK, THURSDAY, AUGUST 4, 1927.          TWO CENTS

# Sacco and Vanzetti Must Die, Says Fuller; Decision Is Backed by His Inquiry Committee

*The evidence of Col Goddard from the Bureau of Forensic Ballistics put paid to any suspicion that Sacco and Vanzetti were innocent (John Frost Historical Newspaper Service).*

both were charged with robbery and murder. Their case was not helped by the presiding judge, the patently biased Webster Thayer. The first trial lasted a fortnight, with the Massachusetts police chief doubling as firearms expert; both men were found guilty – Sacco of murder, Vanzetti as an accessory – and were sentenced to death.

The following day the world's press carried the news in bold headlines, and international left-wing organizations began to clamour for a re-trial, setting up funds for the defence. As a result the executions were postponed while the defence sought further evidence and pressed motion after motion for a fresh hearing. Throughout, the sentenced men steadfastly maintained their innocence.

Finally, in June 1927, Governor Alvin Fuller of Massachusetts yielded to world opinion, and appointed an independent committee under Lawrence Lowell, President of Harvard, to re-examine the whole case. At this point, Colonel Goddard came forward. He explained to both the prosecution and the defence that he had been watching the proceedings with interest; over the past two years he had been carrying on the research work begun by Waite, Fischer and Gravelle and he was now confident that he could bring unbiased scientific evidence to bear. Given the alleged murder weapons and bullets, he would show whether or not they had come from Sacco's revolver. The guilt or innocence of the parties was, of course, another matter.

The defence refused to be associated with Goddard, but the prosecution took up his offer. Armed with helixometer and comparison microscope, Colonel Goddard made his examination, and then showed the committee the evidence. Without doubt, Parmenter and Berardelli had both been killed by shots from Sacco's gun.

When the Lowell Committee reported on Goddard's conclusive evidence, Governor Fuller refused to commute the sentences. On 23 August 1927, the two men went to the chair in Charlestown. Vanzetti's last words were: 'I am innocent'. Sacco, more defiant, cried: 'Long live anarchy'.

The controversy did not stop there. Judge Thayer in particular suffered the consequences of his decision for the rest of his life, with bombs and stones being periodically hurled at him. Over 30 years later two American ballistics experts decided to recheck Goddard's evidence with the more sophisticated modern comparison microscope. In October 1961 they announced their verdict – Goddard had been absolutely right in every detail of his findings. If Vanzetti was possibly innocent, Sacco was not.

Goddard went from strength to strength after the Sacco-Vanzetti affair. Two years later he was able to identify the two Thompson .45 calibre sub-machine guns used in the notorious St Valentine's Day massacre of 1929, when the Capone gang attacked and killed seven members of the rival Bugs Moran outfit. One gun was a stick magazine type with a 20-round capacity, the other a drum type which carried 50 rounds. All 70 bullets were used to riddle the victims.

This particular piece of research impressed J. Edgar Hoover, the young director of the Federal Bureau of Investigation. He and Dr Herman N. Bundesden, the Chicago coroner, urged Goddard to leave New York and set up shop in Chicago, where his services could, for the time being at least, be most useful. As a result Goddard became founder and first director of the Scientific Crime Detection Laboratory at Northwestern University, Evanston, Illinois, which remains one of America's leading crime research centres. And because of the laboratory's success, Hoover set up the FBI Ballistics Department in Washington, today the largest and perhaps busiest forensic ballistics centre in the world.

America was not to have all the plaudits however. Within

months of the Sacco-Vanzetti affair coming to its end two rather less sensational cases had added new facets to criminal ballistics. Both involved a burly English gunmaker in his late thirties named Robert Churchill, who helped cut the umbilical cord which still tied European ballistics to its medico-legal parent.

Churchill was already famous as a sporting gunmaker in the 1920s, with a shop near Leicester Square which was patronized by rich and titled clients. Like Smith, Churchill read about the Waite-Gravelle comparison microscope and sailed for America to see the instrument at first hand. He arrived in 1926, too late to meet Waite, but in good time to be impressed by Goddard. He returned to England with a comparison microscope of his own. Churchill was a friend of Bernard Spilsbury and shared the same fault: once his mind was made up about a case, nothing could change it. As Smith observed, in court – where they were frequently to appear together – they were an impressive team, frightening when they were wrong. Fortunately, most of the time they were right.

On a moonlit night in October 1927, shortly after Churchill's return from America, a 35-year-old labourer named Enoch Dix took his .410 single barrelled shotgun to Whistling Copse, on the estate of Lord Temple near Bath, in Somerset. Dix was a known poacher, and he was recognized instantly by Lord Temple's head keeper, William Walker, and the underkeeper George Rawlings when they hurried to the scene with their twelve bores after hearing his first shots. As the two men arrived Dix spun round and his gun went off; Walker fell dying, while Rawlings took a pot shot at the fleeing poacher.

When the police searched Dix's cottage they found the .410 and ordered its owner to strip. Dix's back and thighs were pitted with pellet wounds; Dix claimed that Rawlings had fired at him first, and his own gun had discharged accidentally with the shock.

Churchill was called in and was faced with the question: who had fired first, and at what range ? Using the underkeeper's gun and identical cartridges, he fired at a series of white-washed metal plates, varying the range. By studying these and the pattern of the wounds on Dix's back, he concluded that Rawlings had hit the poacher at a range of 15 yards; most of the charge, fortunately for Dix, having hit a tree. Therefore if Dix's gun had gone off accidentally, as he claimed, it must have felled Walker at the same range. But shot from Dix's .410 spread to between 27 and 30 inches at 15 yards, whereas the wound in Walker's throat was five inches in diameter. Churchill showed that such a wound could only be produced by Dix's gun at a range of less than five yards – point blank, in fact.

It was a simple piece of calculation – but its like had not been produced as evidence before.

Churchill's second innovative case began exactly a month previous to the Dix affair. On the morning of 27 September, Police Constable George Gutteridge was found shot to death on a lonely road near Stapleford Abbots, Essex. It was a particularly gruesome killing, for besides the two shots which killed the officer he had been shot twice more, through each eye, as he lay on the ground. The motive for this piece of butchery seemed to be superstition; it was still believed by some criminals that the eyes of a murdered man registered the last sight they ever saw photographically.

Some miles away, police found a stolen car with human blood on the running board and an empty .455 cartridge under the driving seat. The following January, acting on information, they arrested a criminal named Frederick Browne, who ran a garage in Brixton with another ex-convict named William Kennedy. On Browne's premises were found a .455 Webley revolver with a quantity of ammunition of the same calibre; moreover the bullets were of rare, obsolete types known as Mark I and Mark IV. Kennedy was arrested a few days later and on 23 April 1928 the pair were tried for murder at the Old Bailey. Churchill led a team of three War Office experts as witnesses and told the court of the research he had carried out on the case.

Firstly, the cartridge found in the stolen car had borne marks identical with those made by the breech face of Browne's Webley. This evidence alone would seem conclusive, but Churchill's men made sure. They test fired no less than 1300 identical revolvers to see if the breech tooling marks could be duplicated in any way. None matched. Furthermore, they showed that the striations on the bullets taken from the body of P.C. Gutteridge matched those on test shots from Browne's weapon. Finally, they pointed out that Mark IV ammunition was loaded with black powder (smokeless powder had replaced this gunpowder in the 1880s), and distinctive black powder marks had surrounded the officer's wounds. It was the first time that forensic ballistics evidence had ever been produced at the Old Bailey, and it was triumphant. Browne and Kennedy went to the gallows.

The Gutteridge case had further-reaching consequences than even the Sacco-Vanzetti verdict on observers on the Continent; within months, ballistics laboratories had been set up in Lyons, Stuttgart, Oslo and Berlin, with Moscow following suit shortly afterwards. At last, forensic ballistics was established worldwide.

# Chapter Five
# Every bullet has its billet

But yet I hadde alway a Coltes tooth,
Gat-toothed I was, and that becam me weel.

Chaucer, *Prologue of the Wyves Tale of Bath*

Despite all Charles E. Waite's dedication to collecting firearms data, his task, in real terms, was an impossible one. The great criminal scientist A. Lucas pointed out the difficulties in his *Forensic Chemistry*:

No matter how comprehensive lists of collections of firearms might be, and even if they included an example of all the weapons made by manufacturers of repute and of all the weapons made by large scale manufacturers of cheap weapons, they would not and could not include examples of the large number of weapons put together by small makers of cheap firearms in different parts of the world, much less examples of the occasional weapon assembled from parts of others by a private 'gunsmith' and still less examples of all amateur-made weapons.

One self-evident fact is that the firearms examiner must be familiar with guns of every type, and to become so is no mean task, for the variety of firearms available is enormous. Roughly speaking, however, they subdivide into several categories, the most obvious being between smooth-bore and the rifled types. Apart from antique weapons, most smooth-bore guns are 'shot' guns which utilize cartridges of cardboard or plastic stopped at one end by a metal percussion cap and at the other by a cardboard wad. They are filled with powder and a charge of small lead pellets.

Although there are automatic and pump action repeating shotguns available, most are single- or double-barrelled, with one cartridge for each barrel; the barrels are usually hinged to the stock and the cartridges are loaded into the breech and ejected by hand after firing. One or both barrels may be 'choked' at the muzzle end – restricted to give a narrower shot pattern;

when fired, the lead pellets leave the gun as a mass, but spread apart over a given distance, and, as in the Dix case quoted in the previous chapter, experts can determine the distance of the gun from the target by examining the impact of the shot and measuring its spread. As with the case of other firearms, the breech-block and firing pin of a shotgun leave their mark on the fired cartridge.

At close range the shotgun is a devastating weapon. The 'sawn-off' shotgun with the barrels cut down to a few inches and the stock shortened to pistol grip size is for convenience only; at point-blank range it will inflict a hideous wound, but the fast spread of shot from the stumpy barrels quickly renders it less lethal.

Of the rifled variety of firearms there are many, ranging from machine guns and sub-machine guns through automatic rifles, bolt action rifles, revolvers, and the so-called 'automatic' pistols. With the passing of the Capone era, machine and sub-machine guns have become less common in crime, though they are favoured, along with rifles, by political assassins and 'hit' men, anxious to kill from a distance and make a swift getaway. The revolver and the 'automatic', easily hidden and portable, are the favourite weapons of the average criminal. Of the two, most experts would argue that the revolver, with a more robust build and less of a tendency to jam, is the more reliable.

Most American police forces today are armed with the Smith & Wesson .38 revolver. One of Smith & Wesson's earliest guns was the .44 Model 1870, popularly known as the 'American'. The 'American' was a hinged frame pistol – the barrel opened downwards to give access to the chambers for loading – and was fitted with the Dodge & King ejector system in which a central star-shaped plate moved out from the rear of the cylinder when the weapon was 'broken' open, forcing out the empty cartridges. The 'American' became popular on both sides of the law – both Wyatt Earp and Jesse James carried one – and aspects of it have continued in production in other models today. Most importantly for criminologists, the star plate ejector, like other ejector systems, leaves its mark on the end of the cartridges and helps in identification.

There is a story that the Russians, shortly after the introduction of the 'American', sent a military deputation to the United States in search of new weaponry. While there, the general in charge went on a hunting trip with 'Buffalo Bill' Cody and was much taken by Cody's 'American'. As a result he ordered nearly a quarter of a million modified .44s which became known as the '.44 Russian'. At least one of these was used in the assassination of the Russian Royal Family after the revolution of 1917.

The modern Smith & Wesson 'police' .38 is a solid frame pistol which is loaded by releasing a catch and swinging out the entire cylinder on a hinge to the left for loading. It is considered to be a 'humane' gun, in that an expert marksman can 'wing' a fugitive without killing him.

Apart from the usual breech face and firing pin marks, the 'swing out' type of revolver such as the Smith & Wesson .38 leaves no ejector marks on its cartridges simply because no ejector is fitted; it does leave scope for the fingerprint expert, however, because in the case of tight fitting cartridges the shells cannot be shaken out and have to be pulled out between finger and thumb, as is the case with most shotgun shells. Thus a good thumb print may possibly be left – thumb prints planted during loading are, of course, destroyed by the cartridge being slammed against the breech block during firing.

Only the rod ejector system in revolvers – a comparative rarity nowadays – leaves little or no mark and yet enables its operator to empty the chamber without leaving his prints on the shells. The Colt Model 1873 – the 'Frontier' or 'Peacemaker' – uses rod ejection, and because of this and other factors can present peculiar problems in a murder investigation.

The 'Frontier' is a 'single action' revolver; the operator thumbs back the hammer to cock it and then pulls the trigger, whereas in a double action pistol like most in use today a single pull on the trigger cocks the hammer and drops it in one. The 'Frontier' is loaded by thumbing open a 'gate' to the right of the hammer which gives access to each of the six chambers in turn. The spring loaded ejector rod lies along the right side of the barrel, and when firing is completed the gate is again opened and the rod pushed back to poke out the cartridges.

It is not as robust as its contemporary, the Smith & Wesson

American, but the Frontier has other advantages, despite the tendency of its rather delicate mechanism to break down, the chief one being that it is possible to fire the gun under almost any conditions. If the trigger spring breaks, a single shot can be fired by thumbing the hammer in the ordinary way and letting it slip. It is possible, if necessary, to 'fan' all six shots, given a certain dexterity, by turning the cylinder with the right thumb while slapping back the hammer with the heel of the left hand: many Hollywood desperados preferred this method anyway, although it would seem impossible to achieve any accuracy. Finally, if the mainspring – the spring which operates the hammer – breaks, it is still possible to point the gun and bang the spur of the hammer with something heavy to strike the cartridge. In fact it was its very ease of firing, even in perfect condition, which led professional gunmen to load the six-shooter with only five bullets, letting the hammer rest on the empty chamber so as to avoid blowing off a foot when the gun was holstered. If a gunman habitually 'carried five beans in the wheel' he knew his business.

The Colt Frontier is still in the forefront of American crime – and still causes headaches to ballistics experts – because of its ubiquity. It was produced continually from 1873 to 1941 and then, after a break, from 1955 until the present day. From 1873 to 1891 it was the standard side arm of the United States Army, some 36,000 being delivered, all with seven and a half inch barrels and all in .45 calibre. It was this latter fact that gave the Frontier its popular appellation 'Colt .45' – which is misleading, not only because the company have produced numerous other .45 models, but because the original Frontier was probably most popular among cattlemen and lawmen in the .44-40 calibre. It has, in fact, been produced in almost every calibre from .22 rimfire to .476 Eley. One of the most up to date versions – changed only in barrel and cylinder size – loads the massive .357 Magnum.

The successor to the Colt .45 revolver with the United States Army since the First World War has been another version of the Colt .45, this time a self-loading weapon of the type popularly and erroneously known as an 'automatic'.

Properly speaking a true automatic gun is one which begins to fire when the trigger is pressed and carries on until either the magazine is empty or the trigger pressure is removed. Into this category come the various types of modern automatic rifle which can either fire one shot or a burst, sub-machine guns such as the familiar Thompson drum-magazine weapon used by G men and gangsters during Prohibition – the 'Chicago piano' – and the war-time Sten, as well as the heavier machine guns used in tanks and aircraft.

The self-loading pistol fires one shot at a time with each pull of the trigger, but it is a vastly more complex weapon than the revolver, almost every model having minute variations in its interior mechanism. Basically, the average 'automatic' consists of an oblong frame with a hollow handle into which the long metal magazine is inserted after being loaded with its complement of rounds – often nine, twelve or more. (The heaviest load of any handgun is 14.) On top of the frame lies the barrel and barrel-extension, which is covered by a long slide containing the spring loaded bolt with its firing pin – the Colt 'automatic' in fact, like several others, has an external hammer like that of a revolver which can be cocked manually.

The user takes the pistol in the hand he favours and grips the rear of the slide with the forefinger and thumb of his other hand, drawing it back towards him. This causes a bullet to be extracted from the magazine, and cocks the firing pin; when he releases the slide the bullet is forced into the breech. He then presses the trigger. We have already seen that tremendous pressure is exerted in a 'blow back' fashion on a cartridge in any gun being fired, and it is this pressure which now forces back the slide a microsecond after the bullet has left the gun. The retraction of the slide activates an ejector mechanism which throws the spent cartridge out through an aperture to the right of the pistol, and then the slide travels forward as before, picking the next round from the magazine and slotting it into the breech. The gun is now cocked and loaded, ready for firing again.

Because of all this mechanical action the 'automatic' is perhaps the most popular weapon of all with firearms examiners, for besides marks from the firing pin and ejector, traces are also left on the metal of the cartridge by the magazine, slide, bolt face, chamber wall, and extractor. But, as has been stated before, the very complexity of the self-loading pistol detracts from its reliability.

In 1974 a fanatic attempted to kidnap Princess Anne, travelling with her husband and her customary armed Special Branch man through London towards Buckingham Palace. The would-be kidnapper forced the Royal automobile to a stop at gun point, whereupon the Special Branch officer drew his Walther 7.65 mm automatic, and in a split second of horror found that it had jammed. Both he and a passer-by who stopped were wounded before the gunman was finally over-powered. Police officers had only recently been issued with the Walther, which supplanted the traditional British Webley .38 revolver for bodyguard duties. The Walther 7.65 mm seemed to have all the advantages over the older weapon; it is slim and relatively light at 1 lb 5 oz fully loaded with seven shots, and has a muzzle velocity of 950 feet per second. The Webley, on the other hand, a bulky standard six-shot pistol, weighs 1 lb 11 oz, with a muzzle velocity of 600 feet per second.

'But,' as one senior police officer remarked scathingly after the kidnap attempt, 'you could rely on the awkward beast. The bloody thing never jammed.'

If anything, the question of true 'ballistics' – the study of cartridges – is more complex than the study of firearms themselves; for every pistol of every calibre in existence there are at least a dozen different makes and patterns of cartridge available. In the United States, Britain, and many of the Commonwealth countries, rifled arms are classified by calibre, this is the distance across the internal diameter of the bore between the lands, measured in decimal points of an inch. On the Continent, the same measurement is registered in millimetres.

Even then, the question of calibre is a complex one. A .45 round for instance may be very long (as used in the Colt Peacemaker) or it may be a soft nosed 'short' round with a relatively low muzzle velocity. Either the bullet or the cartridge case may be shorter or longer according to purpose, and may be designed for firing from a revolver or from an automatic.

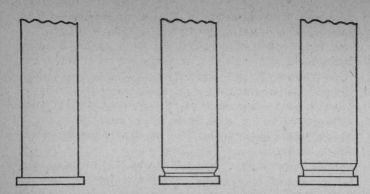

Rimmed cartridge case  Semi-rimmed cartridge case  Rimless cartridge case

*Revolvers and shotguns take rimmed cartridges, while most 'automatics' are loaded with the rimless variety.*

Cartridges may be rimmed, semi-rimmed, or rimless. Most rimmed cartridges are designed for shotguns or revolvers, the rim being designed to fit around the base of the cylinder or chamber cone to stop the shell sliding through. In a 'rim fire' cartridge, the primer to be hit by the hammer is contained in the rim itself.

The rare semi-rimmed cartridge is used in certain self-loading pistols, but most 'automatic' rounds are usually rimless; instead they have a groove which runs around the circumference of the base and gives the ejector a grip on the spent shell. All cartridge cases may be either straight sided or 'bottle necked' where the round is smaller in diameter than the case itself; these are usually for rifles.

The bullets themselves come in a variety of shapes and designs. There are ball bullets, almost spherical in shape, ogival or round-nosed bullets, truncated or flat-nosed bullets, and bullets with hollow points. They may be smooth-surfaced or have one or more canelures or grooves cut into them, and they may be plain lead or cupro-nickel jacketed with a filling of lead, zinc or other metals.

Between the wars the British Army .303 rounds were composed of a cartridge packed with cordite, as a propellant, and a compound bullet consisting of a cupro-nickel jacket with an inner tip of aluminium backed by a slug of lead. Investigating the mass shooting of rioters in Egypt during the twenties, Professor Sir Sydney Smith recovered a number of bullets and discovered that, in some of them, paper pulp had been used in place of the aluminium tip. Accordingly, he wrote to the War Office in London reporting the fact and suggesting first that some contractor was using paper pulp as a substitute for aluminium and secondly that it seemed to fulfil the same function as the aluminium.

Smith received the reply that the paper pulp had been used in .303 ammunition after the supply of aluminium gave out during the First World War. He was assured that the light metal tip

. . . conferred on the bullet certain ballistic advantages which were not disclosed to me but which were, I was assured, invaluable. Nor, said the War Office, was I right in thinking that it would be cheaper to use paper than aluminium, for the pulp had to be put through several processes and thoroughly sterilized so that wound infection should not take place.

This, wrote Smith, struck him as an 'exceedingly delicate thoughtfulness for the victims of the shooting' – not unlike attempts after the Second World War to develop a 'clean' nuclear weapon. Whether it was misguided delicacy or not is for moralists to judge, for the Russians possibly, and the Germans certainly, developed a poisonous bullet during the Second World War, though whether it ever went into service is doubtful.

It was a version of the highly successful 9 mm Parabellum cartridge, developed as an ordinary round in about thirty different variations. The 9 mm Kampstoff-Patrone 08 contained an unusual bullet with a nose cavity and channel cut into its lead core, a capsule of potassium cyanate, and a steel 'after-core'. The jacket was of thin steel. The idea was that the steel after-core flew forward when the bullet hit its target and smashed the capsule against the lead bullet core, ejecting the poison through the core channel. This seems to have been gilding the lily somewhat, for the ordinary 9 mm Parabellum was quite capable of killing without any poison being added.

Poison and ballistics came together only once in forensic history, and that in a case which, had it succeeded, would have been as controversial in its day as the J. F. Kennedy assassination; that it did not was due to the incompetence of its planners, rather than the methods proposed. In March 1917, British Military Intelligence received a report of a strange group operating in Derby. Its members consisted of a certain Mrs Wheeldon, her son-in-law, who was a chemist from Southampton, and her two daughters. Coupled with the Wheeldon group were a variety of political malcontents, conscientious objectors, pro-German sympathizers, and 'bolsheviks'. It was a curious admixture, and the head of anti-subversion at Military Intelligence, Major Melville Lee, sent an agent named Gordon to Derby to infiltrate the group. Posing as an anarchist, Gordon soon gained admittance to the Wheeldon organization, whose watchword, he reported, was 'Lloyd George must die'. Lloyd George was then Prime Minister.

Major Lee was inclined to take Gordon's report seriously. Only one British Prime Minister, Spencer Perceval in 1812, has ever been assassinated in office, and he was killed by a madman rather than a political opponent, but there was no point in taking chances. Lee now sent a second agent, Herbert Booth, to Derby. Booth gained access as easily as Gordon had done, posing as an Army deserter who had been a crack-shot. Unwittingly, his story fitted in with the plans of the Wheeldon group perfectly. Mrs Wheeldon handed him a powerful air-rifle and several darts coated with curare; he was to lie in wait for the Prime Minister at his favourite golf course, Walton Heath, and shoot him down from hiding. The almost silent air-gun would allow him to escape without difficulty. To keep his darts in good condition Booth was handed an extra two tubes of curare, sent to his mother-in-law by the chemist, who also supplied two tubes of strychnine containing nine grains – a quarter of a grain can be a fatal dose.

Armed with this evidence, Booth contacted Major Lee and the whole group were arrested. Scientific evidence given at the trial showed that the plot could have succeeded. Curare when mixed with water forms a sticky substance long used by South American tribes to coat their arrows. It can be swallowed without ill effect, but when introduced into a wound paralyses first the motor nerve endings of the spinal column and then the respiratory system, causing asphyxia.

It was probably the incompetence of the plot which determined the relatively light sentences handed out to Mrs Wheeldon and her son-in-law the chemist. She received ten years hard labour, he seven, but Lloyd George, who appears to have treated the whole affair as a joke, soon afterwards procured their release from jail.

Much is made of the hitting power of the modern Magnum ammunition, and it is true that a hand-gun heavy and strong enough to take this highly charged type of cartridge can be formidable. Perhaps the most powerful hand-gun in the world today, with the Ruger Blackhawk, is the .44 Magnum Smith & Wesson Model 29, which was produced specifically to chamber the Remington .44 Magnum cartridge in the late 50s. At 2 lb 14 oz it is a heavy gun, as it needs to be to soak up the massive recoil, akin, as one expert puts it 'to touching off a howitzer single-handed'.

The bullet leaves the muzzle of the pistol at 1540 feet per second – over four hundred feet per second faster than sound – and as it does so it develops 'tail wag'. Tail wag happens in all rifled weapons, and is similar to the wobble of a child's top before it settles into steady motion. At close range this tail wag makes an entrance hole much bigger than the bullet itself, and exits with proportionally wider effect.

But tail wag is far greater in a rifle, which has an even higher velocity than a hand-held Magnum. The average high-powered rifle has a muzzle velocity of at least 2,500 feet per second, sometimes much more, and when the bullet leaves it, it is spinning at between two and three thousand revolutions per second. Even when its tail wag has steadied, its impact on a resistant surface is curious, for the cupro-nickel jacket often turns inside out, like a glove being pulled off a hand. At the same time there is a splash-back effect which gives the entrance the appearance of an exit hole. If the bullet is still unsteady – at up to three or four hundred yards – its impact may create the effect of a small explosion.

Tests show that if a high velocity bullet is fired into soft clay it does not pass straight through; the pressure it carries creates a huge cavity far larger than the projectile itself, and often the bullet is smashed to pieces. Wounds at such ranges often look like the effect of dum-dum or exploding bullets. They may also lead the inexperienced firearms examiner to the impression that more than one shot has been fired, as a curious case which occurred in Edinburgh in 1940 showed.

At midnight on 12 July, a police car containing the Assistant Chief Constable of the city, along with three other officers, was travelling towards the city centre during an air raid alert. The Assistant Chief Constable was sitting beside the driver while the other two officers were in the back. Suddenly, a Royal Air Force sergeant stepped into the road and challenged the driver to stop. The driver did not do so and as the vehicle passed by the sergeant fired his .303 rifle through the celluloid of the rear window and hit the Assistant Chief Constable on the chin. The car stopped and, with the sergeant handcuffed to one of the officers in the back, the car was driven at high speed to the Royal Infirmary, for the senior officer had suffered a massive face wound. He died some time later.

At the autopsy, it was discovered that the bullet had entered cleanly just behind the chin on the right and then disintegrated. The lower jaw was completely shattered, and the exit wound, about three and a half inches wide, stretched from the jaw line up to the level of the ear, with the flesh and bone fragments bursting outward. It appeared that the bullet had merely touched the bone but that its velocity and tail wag had caused disintegration not only of the whole jaw but of the bullet itself, for fragments were found in the mouth and skull.

When ballistics experts examined the car, they were convinced that at least two or three shots must have been fired at it. Apart from the entrance hole in the rear window, there were what appeared to be two separate bullet holes in the licence holder and the windscreen, while another projectile appeared to have exited through the door-frame to the Assistant Chief Constable's left. On the upper edge of the windscreen frame was an oval dent about an inch in length which bore traces of cupro-nickel, and the woodwork of the dashboard had been peppered with small fragments of embedded lead, nickel and human bone. On the back seat, the aluminium tip and cupro-nickel jacket of a .303 was found.

Despite this evidence the three surviving police officers said that only one shot had been fired, and examination of the airman's rifle seemed to prove this; the magazine contained only three rounds, although it had a five-round capacity, the fourth was in the breech, while a spent .303 cartridge was found at the scene of the crime.

A reconstruction of the crime, using the actual vehicle and blank bullets, showed that even a skilled rifleman could not have fired at the car, worked the bolt of his rifle and hit the car again in such a way as to cause the interior markings at the speed the vehicle was travelling. So one bullet had done all the damage.

If the rear window had been glass instead of celluloid, the high velocity bullet with its low speed wobble might well have disintegrated on impact there; instead it took the slightly firmer but still ludicrously fragile structure of a human jaw bone to cause the strongly cased bullet to explode. The flying fragments still had sufficient force to pierce the metal of the door frame and the licence holder, as well as the windscreen. The largest piece – the bullet tip – had apparently hit the windscreen frame before rebounding into the back seat, missing the other occupants of the car. Interestingly, the firearms experts noted that, instead of going forward in the direction of the discharge from the rifle – from right to left and slightly downward – it had struck the jaw-bone and flown off at an acute angle, upward and from left to right, showing the danger in assuming that any fragment of bullet that disintegrates will necessarily continue in the same line of flight as when leaving the gun.

The sergeant was brought to trial on a charge of assault and culpable homicide, and in his defence claimed that he had been acting on instructions from an unnamed senior officer to challenge cars travelling during the air raid. Evidence was given

105

that he had been drinking before the incident, and because of this and his good service record he was given a mere six months' imprisonment.

Two cases reported by Sir Sydney Smith are worth quoting here as an example of the difficulties which may face a medico-legal examiner and firearms examiner in judging the number of shots and direction of fire. In the first, an Army deserter was involved in a fire-fight at close range and was hit at a distance of about ten to fifteen yards with a service rifle. The bullet passed through both legs, and the man died shortly afterwards from haemorrhage.

When Smith examined the body he noted that the bullet had entered the outer side of the left thigh, and the entrance wound was clean cut and characteristic. The bullet traversed the fleshy part of the thigh, passing behind the femur, and although the great vessels were undamaged the muscle was pulped. This muscle damage increased as the track approached the exit, which was made on the inner side of the thigh. The exit hole was two and a half inches in diameter, with scraps of tissue and muscle forced out of it.

The bullet had then entered the inner side of the right thigh, leaving a lacerated wound three by six inches in size. After destroying skin and fibrous tissue and pulping more muscle the bullet struck the lower end of the femur, powdering it, and tearing the femoral artery and nerve; a few fragments of the bullet tore a small hole in the outside of the right thigh. It was evident that the bullet had broken up in the right thigh muscle before it hit the bone.

'Anyone without experience or knowledge of the circumstances of the shooting might, on looking at the wounds, have assumed that two shots had been fired, one from the left and the other from the right,' reported Sir Sydney.

In another freakish case, a young soldier was badly wounded in all four limbs, and each had an entrance and exit wound. When the injured man was taken to hospital even Sir Sydney, with his inbred caution about matters of ballistics, considered that four bullets must have been fired. In fact it transpired that the soldier had been bending down to adjust his puttees when a comrade's Lewis gun accidentally went off at a range of about a yard. The bullet entered the outer side of his left leg below the knee, came out on the inner side and entered his left arm below the elbow, went through that and then through his right leg, and finally passed through his right arm.

'One of the interesting features of this case,' Sir Sydney wrote, 'was that the bullet did comparatively little damage in the first three limbs, and only exploded and disintegrated after striking the bone in the right arm.'

To add to the difficulties facing investigators where massive wounds are concerned, small calibre explosive bullets have been experimented with from time to time. The 'dum dum' mentioned previously was a favourite on the Afghan frontier and was also used extensively in Egypt. It was simply an ordinary bullet with a cross-shaped cut in the nose, and caused the same effect as a high velocity bullet when fired from a low velocity weapon. The idea was taken a stage further during World War Two, again by the Germans, and again in an adaptation of the 9 mm Parabellum. A pellet of lead azide – a sensitive and powerful detonator – was placed under high pressure in the bullet's nose. Inert when pressurized, the pellet was supposed to explode when the pressure was released on impact. The cartridge was termed the 9 mm Sprengpatrone 08 but its explosive capacity and potential were small. Again, a case of gilding the lily.

Of course, whether a bullet explodes 'naturally' or otherwise, it presents problems to the ballistics expert. If the fragments are small – and they usually are – it is virtually impossible to examine them for rifling marks, and, as the case of the Edinburgh policeman shows, direction of fire is difficult to judge. But when shots come from a low powered weapon it is usually possible, by measuring the angles of the wounds, to give a precise indication of the position of the attacker and the attacked at the time of the assault. Sir Bernard Spilsbury produced succinct evidence to this effect at the trial of two IRA men convicted of gunning down Field Marshal Sir Henry Wilson in 1922. Sir Henry, formerly Chief of the Imperial General Staff, was an Irishman who served as Member of Parliament for North Down and was a supporter of the partition between Northern and Southern Ireland. After one visit to Ulster, where he had made himself unpopular with Republicans by advising on the policing of the new border, he returned to London and on the morning of 22 June unveiled a war memorial at Liverpool Street station. Returning home to Eaton Place in full dress uniform, complete with sword, he had paid his taxi and was feeling for his keys when two men came up behind him, drew revolvers, and began firing. As the first two shots hit him he tried to draw his sword but seven more bullets hit him in rapid succession and he fell dying on his own doorstep. With their three remaining bullets his attackers wounded three of their captors before being arrested.

Spilsbury carried out his first examination of Wilson's body as the dead man lay on a couch in his drawing room. He had been shot in the left forearm, twice in the right arm, twice in the left shoulder, in both armpits, and twice in the right leg; the armpit wounds extended through to the lungs and had been fatal. On this way out, Spilsbury made calculations from bullet marks in the front door, and then made his report. He wrote,

Wilson was not shot after he had fallen. All nine wounds were inflicted when he was erect or slightly stooping, as he would be when tugging at his sword hilt. The chest injuries were from shots fired at two different angles – one from right to left and the other from left to right. Either would have proved fatal and produced death inside ten minutes. The bullet through the right leg passed forwards and downwards, and therefore the shot came from directly behind. That in the top left shoulder had been fired from the left side and rather behind, and the downward direction proved that the arm was in a raised position as the bullet entered. The wounds in the forearms were inflicted from behind whilst the arms were still at the side of the body.

The two men, Connolly and O'Brien, were hanged.

Besides the evidence offered by bullets, particles of bullets, cartridge cases, and the weapons themselves, the firearms examiner has other details to attend to when a firearms offence is committed. He works, of course, with the pathologist in the case of murder, and where possible will visit the victim of a serious wounding as soon as possible after the crime is committed. Where powder deposits are found at the scene or on the victim or his clothing, the forensic chemist is brought in, but powder burns or 'tattooing' on the skin of the victim are also measured by the firearms examiner. The extent of these can sometimes show the range of fire with accuracy if the murder weapon is available. Powder burns have, in fact, been detected around a wound caused by a shot from a yard away.

Until recently, ballistics departments in both the United States and Britain were responsible for conducting a 'dermal nitrate test' on anyone recently suspected of firing a gun. The idea was that the burned powder produces nitrates which are blown back from the muzzle of a weapon when it is fired, and these invisibly stain the hand of the marksman. Unfortunately nitrates are also deposited on the hands of cigarette and cigar smokers, as well as people who have handled chemicals such as fertilizers; the dermal nitrate test is therefore now realized to be unreliable and has been almost universally discontinued.

In its stead, swabs are taken from the suspect's hands and compared with those lifted from the victim's wounds and clothing and are tested for the presence of two elements, lead and barium. Sodium rhodizinate, which is specific for both metals, is used as a reagent, but even this test is usually used to eliminate a suspect rather than supply evidence of involvement.

However, experiments are still going on in determining the presence of cartridge residue on the hands of a suspect, for 'blow back' evidence seems too good to waste. Blow back always occurs when a revolver is fired, usually where a self-loading pistol or shotgun is concerned, and sometimes where a rifle not in first rate condition has been used.

Warm melted paraffin is poured over the suspect's hand, set, and then peeled off to form a kind of thin skinned glove. This glove is then placed in the heart of a nuclear reactor until it is radio-active and thus gives off gamma rays. In a gamma ray spectrometer, the scientist sorts and measures the wavelengths of the rays to show what elements are present. If mercury, lead, antimony or barium are present, the chances are that the suspect has recently fired a gun; but it is only fair to say that when this process was tried on Lee Harvey Oswald, President Kennedy's assassin, all the results were negative.

A popular feature of detective fiction has the examiner lifting a pistol to his nose, sniffing it, and pronouncing that it has been recently fired. Unfortunately, unless this is done within minutes of the firing, in real life it tells the investigator nothing. If the gun has been in regular use – a farmer's shotgun, say – and has not been cleaned recently, the smell of powder will remain strong. The use of the helixometer may give more definite clues, but the firearms examiner will also want to know the history of the weapon immediately after firing – whether it was carried in a pocket or a holster or wrapped in cloth – and will test it for dust and fibre particles. All these can play a part in the build-up of evidence.

A firearms examiner will sometimes question witnesses who saw or heard the shooting, but he will do so with some reserve. The sound waves caused by the discharge of a gun can cause echoes in a confined space which sound like two or more shots, and in the case of the firing of a rifle at more than the speed of sound a second 'shot' will be heard as the bullet breaks the sound barrier. This may well have been the case at the Kennedy assassination, where witnesses 'heard' shots coming both from the Texas Book Depository, and the 'grassy knoll' area to one side. A ricocheting bullet may also 'whine' after the fashion of Western films, further confusing the 'ear-witness'.

As can be seen, the field of forensic ballistics – youngest of all major branches of forensic science – is a vastly complex one, and in each individual case needs a more or less fresh approach. As each new development, however small, occurs, it is exchanged with ballistics centres throughout most parts of the world, and thus the mass of information begun by men like Waite, Goddard, Smith and Churchill continues to build up, as the use of firearms becomes more and more prevalent.

# Chapter Six
# No two alike

Where order in variety we see
And where, though all things differ, all agree.

Alexander Pope, *Windsor Forest*

The problem of identifying offenders against the codes of society has troubled lawmakers since the earliest times. For centuries a negative view was taken; felons were branded or mutilated partly as punishment but also that they might easily be recognized. The biblical injunction to cut off an 'offending' hand is taken literally in parts of the Middle East even today, while liberal Holland was in fact the last country, along with Russia, to abolish branding in the nineteenth century. France abolished the practice after the Revolution, but reintroduced it for a period in the 1930s, while in Ireland the 'pitchcapping' of criminals and political rebels – coating the scalp with molten pitch to leave a permanent, terrible scar – was carried on spasmodically until the 1850s.

In the British Isles and in colonial America, ears were cropped and nostrils slit for relatively trivial offences, while in ancient India the practice of amputating the noses of adulterers became so common that it brought considerable profit to surgeons. The celebrated Hindu anatomist Susruta, writing in the ninth century BC, gives detailed instructions for carrying out rhinoplasty – plastic surgery for rebuilding noses – and, as far as can be judged, his operations were successful.

The first man to take a more positive attitude to the identification of criminals was Eugene Francois Vidocq, who founded the Paris Sûreté in the early years of the nineteenth century. Vidocq's photographic memory covered both facts and faces, and as far as possible he trained his assistants to memorize the personal details of the criminals with whom they dealt. Though he retired in the 1830s, his successors at the Sûreté retained his methods, and they were gradually adopted by the growing law enforcement agencies of Britain and America.

But Vidocq's memory system had an obvious flaw: a 'known' criminal's appearance could be altered, either by accident or design. He could change his hairstyle, grow or shave off a beard, acquire a tattoo or a scar, lose a finger or an eye. And of course, as he grew older his voice, girth, and gait tended to change too.

What criminal records existed were almost unbelievably lax by present day standards; descriptions were restricted to such vague adjectives as 'tall' 'thin' and 'stocky'; and the photographs which accompanied them as the use of the camera spread were easily distorted by the prisoner pulling faces. But as the nineteenth century drew into its middle years, scientists began to look more closely at the basic configurations of the human body. Charles Darwin's *Origin of Species*, published in 1859, sparked off not only rage in the hearts of theologians but excitement in the eager minds of scientists throughout Europe.

Among the latter were Achille Guillard, a well known French naturalist and mathematician, and his son-in-law Dr Louis Adolphe Bertillon, a physician who was also Vice President of the Anthropological Society in Paris. Like the Italian psychiatrist Cesare Lombroso, the two Frenchmen carried out experiments in classifying the shapes and sizes of different skulls of all races, in an attempt to show a relationship between brain size and intellectual achievement. Their studies were watched, without a great deal of interest, by Dr Louis Bertillon's lethargic son Alphonse.

Alphonse Bertillon was a great disappointment to his illustrious father and grandfather; apart from a certain flair for mathematics, his school results were unsatisfactory, and his weak constitution and flat character seemed to make him unfit for any dramatic role in life. After he had been dismissed from his first job in a Paris bank, his father managed to secure him a place as assistant clerk in the records office of the *préfecture de police*.

Young Bertillon's duties involved taking down the particulars of prisoners as they were brought in under arrest, and making out their record cards. He quickly realized that, compared with the painstaking work put in on human measurements by his father and grandfather, the police efforts were pathetic. He also

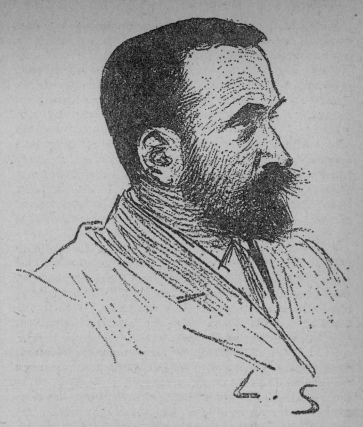

*Alphonse Bertillon, the founder of the system which he named anthropometry, but which was soon known as bertillonage (Mary Evans Picture Library).*

remembered the work being done by his father's friend, the Belgian statistician Lambert Quetelet. Quetelet had suggested that the chances against any two people being the same height were four to one. Working from here, Bertillon reasoned that if only one extra bodily measurement were taken, the chances against two people being equal in both respects were sixteen to one. The odds were lengthened as more measurements were taken: if fourteen measurements were used, he calculated, the odds were 268,435,454 to one.

This theory should be invaluable when applied to policework; if measurements were taken carefully and cross-indexed, the chances of a criminal, once convicted and recorded, going unrecognized if he returned to crime would be so reduced as to be infinitesimal. In October 1879, Bertillon sent a report to this effect to the Prefect of Police, Louis Andrieux. Andrieux, a political appointee with little practical interest in police work and no knowledge of mathematics, passed the report on to Gustave Macé, head of the Sûreté. Macé, a successful detective of the Vidocq school who relied on observation, memory, and instinct, seems to have thought young Bertillon's findings irrelevant and confusing. He turned down the report.

However, Alphonse was now excited for the first time in his life. He appealed to his father for help, and the elder Bertillon immediately saw the basic soundness of his son's idea. After three years of political manipulation, Doctor Louis managed to attract the interest of Andrieux's successor as Prefect, Jean Camecasse, to the system which Alphonse had termed 'anthropometry' – 'man measurement'.

In November 1882, Camecasse agreed to give the young man three months in which to prove his system with a practical demonstration. Elated, Bertillon returned to his office, but as the weeks slipped by his eagerness began to turn to despair. It seemed to him that either his system was malfunctioning or the time limit imposed by the Prefect was going to let him down.

He had begun to file his cards in a cross-indexing system learned from his father. Basically, each measurement was classified as large; medium, or small. If a prisoner with a medium-sized head came in, he would measure the length of the head and then refer back to his collection of cards on file. Should he then find an entry in the medium file whose length corresponded exactly with that of the head under scrutiny, he measured its breadth and checked in the three categories of 'head breadth' file – again large, medium or small. Each tallying measurement led him further through his card system until in theory he was able to say whether or not the incoming prisoner was already 'known'.

By mid-February 1883, Bertillon had 1600 cards on file, but so far none of the prisoners brought in during his rapidly decreasing test period had matched them. But then, late in the afternoon of 20 February, the development he had hoped for occurred.

A prisoner calling himself Dupont was brought in. Bertillon began taking and comparing his measurements, and as he was led through the card system by one corresponding measurement after another, his excitement mounted. Finally he was down to a single card. Stammering, he told 'Dupont' that the police had seen him before. 'You were arrested for stealing empty bottles on December 15 last year. At that time you called yourself Martin.' 'So what?' shrugged the prisoner. 'So I was . . .'

The following day the Paris newspapers published short and unsensational accounts of Bertillon's new system. But Prefect Camecasse was sufficiently impressed to extend Bertillon's time limit, and during the rest of the year he was able to identify nearly 50 recidivists whom Macé and his men had failed to recognize, despite their 'Vidocq' training in observation.

Very gradually, Bertillon's fame spread among French police chiefs, and Camecasse allowed him to take on more assistants and enlarge his department. By the end of 1884 the newspapers had quickened their interest – 300 more prisoners had been identified as having previous records – and had dubbed the new method 'bertillonage', a name which was to pass into criminological jargon. Bertillonage was adopted as standard practice by all French prison governors.

With his system thriving, Bertillon now turned his attention to criminal photography. He improved the 'rogues' gallery' pictures by taking shots of both full face and profile: a practice which continues throughout the world. He also introduced what he termed the 'portrait parlé' or 'speaking likeness', a method of classifying the shapes of noses, eyes, mouths and jaws with precision; the portrait parlé, too, is still in operation and is in fact the basis of the modern 'Identikit' system.

On 1 February 1888, Bertillon was given new headquarters, a

large staff, and the title Director of the Police Identification Service. The French press heralded a new era next day:

Bertillonage is the greatest and most brilliant invention the nineteenth century has produced in the field of criminology. Thanks to a French genius, errors of identification will soon cease to exist not only in France but also in the entire world. Hence judicial error based upon false identification will likewise disappear. Long live Bertillonage! Long live Bertillon!

That these resounding prophecies were painfully premature was to be Alphonse Bertillon's bitter tragedy. But he had one great triumph to come before his downfall.

Since 1878, anarchists and their terror tactics had frightened the people of Europe in a manner which was not to be repeated until the 1960s and 1970s. Germany's Kaiser Wilhelm I was twice fired on in the streets of Berlin, on the second occasion suffering slight wounds from shotgun pellets, and attempts were made on the lives of the Spanish and Italian kings. Both Queen Victoria and the Prince of Wales, later Edward VII, were threatened.

In a series of bomb attacks in Paris in the spring of 1892, the home of the Presiding Judge Benoit, who had previously tried anarchists, was destroyed. The Sûreté learned that the bomb had been planted by a man named Leon Leger, also known as Ravachol. Ravachol was a shadowy figure, described to the Paris police simply as being about five feet four, sallow and dark. To sympathisers with the anarchist cause he was a hero, striking down the aggressors and escaping like a ghost into the night.

But police enquiries revealed that a man calling himself Ravachol had once lived at Saint-Etienne and Monbrison. His real name was Francois Koenigstein and, far from being a high idealist, he was wanted for burglary, grave robbing, strangling an old recluse for his money and beating a shopkeeper to death with a hammer.

What was more important, Koenigstein had been measured by Alphonse Bertillon during one of his early arrests for petty crime, so if Ravachol was ever caught and proved to be the same man as the cowardly murderer, the anarchist cause seemed likely to suffer a blow from which it might never recover.

In March 1892, after a second bombing at the house of the State Prosecutor Bulot, a man fitting the description of Ravachol was arrested for both bomb outrages. Bertillon searched through his file cards and rapidly proved that, in fact, the 'bomber hero' was identical with the wanted criminal Koenigstein. When the news was published it was like a sharp needle to the over-inflated red balloon of anarchy. Bertillon himself was treated like a hero, and awarded the Legion of Honour for his service in ridding France of tyranny. His name swept across Europe and America, and almost every police department in the West temporarily considered bertillonage the great criminological wonder of the world.

Little did Alphonse Bertillon know it – to steal a phrase from the penny dreadful writers of the time – but even as his early struggles bore fruit, the seeds of a new system of criminal identification were germinating in the minds of two Britons, both far away in the East, and these were to grow and strangle bertillonage before it reached its prime.

As a young man of 25, William Herschel, who like Bertillon suffered from a weak constitution, had left England to become an Indian administrative clerk in the district of Hooghly. Irritated by the heat, and his tendency to dysentery and fever, he had lost his temper one day in 1858, shortly after his arrival, with a road builder named Rajadar Konai, who had refused to put his name to a government contract. Herschel had grasped the Indian's hand, slammed it down onto an ink-pad used for rubber stamping forms, and pressed the inky fingers onto the contract. Years later he was to confess that he had no conscious knowledge of what he was doing, apart from the need to get the builder's 'mark' onto paper. But then he began to study the strange loops and lines which the Indian's hand had made. Over the next months, largely to alleviate his boredom, he asked other workers to impress their fingerprints onto paper in the same way.

In 1862 Herschel became involved with paying pensions out of Government funds to Bengalis who had retired from the Indian Army. True to type, the young white sahib found it difficult to distinguish the features of one old sepoy from another; he found he was being quietly swindled. A soldier might come in to Herschel's office, leave his mark, collect his pay, and then send a relative around to collect the money anew. To solve this problem, he again resorted to his ink-pad, requiring each claimant to place his fingerprints on both the paybook and the receipt. By checking these against each other, Herschel quickly discovered that no two prints were alike. When word got around, the fraud came to an end.

Intrigued, Herschel called back certain Indians over a period of years to reprint their hands in his notebooks; he also made records of his own. By 1877 he was able to state categorically, in a letter to the Inspector General of the Prisons of Bengal, that human fingerprints did not change with age; they remained exactly the same and, he suggested, might be of use in criminal records. Like Bertillon, he suffered a disappointment. The Inspector General did not think the idea worth looking into. Two years later Herschel returned to England with his notebooks.

At almost precisely the same time as Herschel's ship was sailing, homeward bound, from Bombay harbour, a Scottish doctor named Henry Faulds, who doubled as physiologist and Presbyterian missionary at Tsukiji Hospital, Tokyo, was looking closely at human handprints which he had found in examples of ancient Japanese pottery. He noticed the same curious twisting patterns as had caught Herschel's eye. He also noted that in certain backward Japanese areas, it was still the custom to 'sign' documents with red or black handprints, and began to wonder whether the natives realized that each man's hand was totally different from that of his fellows; for his research showed that this was true. Primarily, Faulds, who like many of his colonial contemporaries was a scientific dilettante, was interested in proving that fingerprints differed from race to race. His early experiments did not seem to indicate this.

Then, in the summer of 1879, only a few months after he began to collect fingerprints, he became the first man on record to solve crime by means of what he termed 'dactylography' – 'finger-writing'.

A thief who climbed over the whitewashed garden wall of a house in Tokyo had left a sooty handprint on the woodwork. Faulds heard about it and went to inspect the print. He was told that the police had already arrested a suspect, and to the polite amusement of the law officers he took the fingerprints of the arrested man and compared them with those on the wall. They did not tally. Faulds confidently announced that the wrong man had been arrested, and his judgment was vindicated a few days later when a second man was arrested and confessed to the crime. His prints fitted exactly the ones left on the wall.

Some weeks later the Tokyo police asked Faulds to help in a second case of theft. This time, Faulds discovered greasy prints on a piece of porcelain, and coincidence played a part in his amateur investigation. Leafing through his files, he discovered matching prints he had taken from a servant in the area during the course of his experiments. When the man confessed, Faulds realized, like Herschel, that his 'discovery' might have criminological significance. Then, as now, the journal in which gentlemen scientists aired their views was the London magazine *Nature*. Faulds wrote a letter to the editor, outlining his theories, and it was published in October 1880.

When bloody finger marks or impressions on clay, glass, etc. exist, they may lead to the scientific identification of criminals. Already I have had experience in two such cases . . . other cases might occur in medico-legal investigations, as when the hands only of some mutilated victim were found . . . . There can be no doubt as to the advantage of having, besides their photographs, a nature-copy of the forever unchangeable finger furrows of important criminals.

By the time the letter was published, Herschel had arrived back in England, and was naturally chagrined that the other man had pre-empted him after 20 years' study of the subject. He too wrote a letter to *Nature* – but, to be fair to Faulds, the importance of the fingerprints as a method of catching criminals did not seem to have occurred to Herschel. After minor controversy in the pages of the magazine, 'dactyloscopy' was quietly forgotten by almost everyone for the next eight years.

One man who had not forgotten it, however, was one of the most distinguished scientific dilettantes of the era, Sir Francis Galton. Galton, son of a rich Birmingham businessman and cousin of Charles Darwin, was a physician, explorer, geographer and balloonist, but anthropology fascinated him most of all, particularly after the publication of his cousin's book. In the spring of 1888, the Royal Institute of London heard of Alphonse Bertillon's success and decided to send an observer to Paris to see bertillonage in action; they chose Galton, who had already done a great deal of work in the comparison of racial physiques and characteristics.

Galton the scientist was not over-impressed. He wrote:

The incorrectness [of bertillonage] lay in treating the measures of different dimensions of the same person as if they were independent variables, which they are not. For example, a tall man is much more likely to have a long arm, foot, or finger than a short one . . . still the system was most ingenious and very interesting.

What was more interesting, to Galton, was the concept behind bertillonage; the idea of identifying criminals with absolute accuracy. His meeting with Bertillon triggered a memory of the Herschel-Faulds letters in *Nature* eight years before, and on his return to London he contacted Herschel through the magazine. Herschel sent him his collection of fingerprints and notes, and Galton too began collecting prints.

Galton found that neither Herschel nor Faulds had been the first to 'discover' the patterns on human hands – and also, incidentally, those on the soles of the feet. As early as 1684 an individual named Nehemia Grew had noted them, and the English naturalist, Thomas Bewick, had in the late eighteenth century engraved his own handprint on a block and printed it in the books he published. As Faulds had noticed, the Japanese and the Chinese 'signed' pottery with the fingers of the potter. It was in the actual classification of fingerprints that Galton was to become an innovator, for without some simple means of breaking them down into groups they were virtually useless as a means of quick identification.

Pondering this problem, Galton again found that work had already been done on fingerprint types; a Polish pathologist named Johann Purkinje had published a treatise on human skin in the 1830s, in which he had mentioned the various patterns which showed on fingertips: whorls, ellipses, triangles, circles and so on. The trouble was, Galton discovered, such patterns ran into dozens of variations; what he needed was something as simple as Bertillon's 'large, medium' and 'small' classification.

Eventually he discovered that almost every print in his collection featured a triangle, formed where the lines of the various patterns ran together. Some had two or more, and other, rarer ones had no triangle at all. But, decided Galton, these triangles – or 'deltas' as he called them from the Greek letter D – could be described as falling into four basic patterns: 1, no triangle; 2, triangle on left; 3, triangle on right; 4, several triangles.

Like Bertillon, Galton began working out mathematical probabilities. If only one print was taken from each criminal for a file, his four simple classes would soon be inundated and thus unworkable. If all ten were taken, however, they could be subdivided by type into innumerable – and therefore small – classifications. In 1891 he published a paper in *Nature* on his investigations so far and then set to work on a full length book on the subject. Titled *Finger Prints*, it appeared in 1892 and attracted worldwide police attention.

By one of the several coincidences which dot the pioneering history of criminal identification, two practical law men on opposite sides of the globe had formed theories of their own on the subject, and Galton's work came in time to act as a catalyst for those ideas.

The first chronologically – and, many authorities still argue, first in terms of his achievements – was a young police officer named Juan Vucetich, a Serbo-Croat who had emigrated to Argentina in 1884. He joined the Buenos Aires police department, and by the time he was 33, in 1891, he was asked by his superiors to set up a system of bertillonage for the force. Though Vucetich's formal education was small, he had a natural aptitude for mathematics, and a quick grasp of ideas; it is said that only a week after receiving his orders he had a thriving anthropometry department at work. But no sooner was his office under way than his mind was diverted by an article in *La Revue Scientifique;* it was a translation of Galton's article in *Nature.*

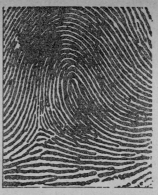

Arches

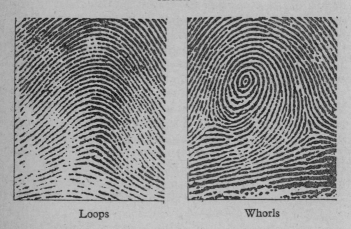

Loops                                          Whorls

*Three basic forms of fingerprint pattern.*

The article had dealt largely with the concept of fingerprints being individual, and had been written too soon to do more than merely outline Galton's struggles with the problems of identification. Vucetich's achievement is thus all the more remarkable: he succeeded in evolving a workable system of classification for fingerprints within a few months.

Apparently independently, he discovered Galton's four basic 'delta' types: no triangles, triangles on the left, triangles on the right, and several triangles. He too classified these, for the fingers, as 1, 2, 3, 4. The same patterns of course, occurred on thumbs, and these he classified as A, B, C, D. Thus he had a working formula for describing the prints of both hands; an example might read C, 1, 4, 4, 2/B, 3, 4, 3, 1.

Vucetich now set up his filing system arranged by letters and numbers; if he wished to check whether a prisoner was already 'known' he simply drew up a ten finger formula and looked in the corresponding file. As his collection grew he saw ways of further sub-classification, and came up with the idea of counting the 'papillary' lines – ridges which make up each print. In July 1892 came the vindication of his efforts, when the Argentine force became the first to solve a crime by means of fingerprinting.

A report came into Buenos Aires headquarters of the shocking murder of two small children, a six-year-old boy and a four-year-old girl, the illegitimate offspring of an attractive young woman named Francisca Rojas. The little family had lived together in a shack in the village of Necochea, and had been visited regularly by a farm labourer named Velasquez, whom the children treated as an uncle, and who was said to be courting Francisca. One night the mother had run screaming incoherently to a neighbour's house with the news that Velasquez had killed her children. The local police were called, and found the children with their heads battered in, lying on their bloodstained bed. Velasquez was arrested, and denied all knowledge of the crime. Questioned by the police, he admitted that he loved Francisca, and had threatened her in an effort to force her into marriage, but he also cared deeply for the children and would never have harmed them.

The Necochea police proceeded to use particularly brutal methods in order to break Velasquez down. First he was beaten almost into insensibility, then revived and tied to the murder bed beside the two corpses and left there all night. The following morning he was near-hysterical, but he persisted in his denial.

The police now discovered that Francisca had another lover, who had offered to marry her if only she could 'get rid of' the children. As a result of this information they resorted to an even more bizarre method of solving the crime; an officer spent all night outside Francisca's hut, knocking on windows and doors and, in sepulchral tones, claimed to be an 'avenging spirit' come to punish the murderer. Francisca emerged the following morning, apparently unmoved by her 'ghostly' experience.

At this point the Necochea police felt that they had come to an impasse, and called in an expert from La Plata headquarters, Inspector Alvarez. Unlike the weird and wonderful methods employed by the local officers, Alvarez's were those of a modern big city officer; he was one of the first policemen to have been impressed by Vucetich's methods. He quickly established that both Velasquez and his rival had alibis covering their whereabouts at the time of the murder; the unfortunate Velasquez, something of a simpleton, had not mentioned the fact to the police in the first place. The most likely culprit, therefore, must be the mother.

Alvarez searched the shack for clues, and came upon a brownish print on the bedroom door. Through his magnifying glass, he saw that it was a human fingerprint, made in what seemed to be blood. The police officer had the print cut from the door in a lump, and took the wood down to Necochea police station. There he asked for an ink-pad and forced Francisca Rojas to imprint her fingers onto a plain sheet of paper. A quick comparison through the magnifying glass showed that the print on the door had been made by the woman's right thumb, and, confronted by this evidence, she broke down and confessed.

Further successes followed: by 1894, the Argentine police had discarded bertillonage and became the first country in the world to adopt 'dactyloscopy' as the sole means of criminal identification. Vucetich spoke of his methods at the Second Scientific Congress of South America in 1901, and by 1908 every country in South America was converted to the science of fingerprinting.

But lack of communication failed to broadcast Vucetich's methods back to Europe – or even to the United States. There, when it came, fingerprinting was to be due to the second man influenced by the works of Sir Francis Galton. He was Edward Henry who, as Inspector General of the Bengal Police, first read Galton's book in 1893.

Bertillonage had come to British India in the early 1890s, and Henry took a keen interest in it. But after hearing of Galton's work he added fingerprints to his anthropometrical files with some success, and while home on leave in 1894 he paid a visit to Galton at his London laboratory. The genial old scientist, now in his seventies, welcomed Henry and placed all his research at his disposal. Back in India, Henry began to work on Galton's half-finished classification system.

Unlike Galton and Vucetich, Henry decided that there were five basic discernible patterns to every set of prints. These he defined as arches A, tented arches T, radial loops R, ulna loops U, and whorls W. Radial loops slope towards the radius bone on the outside of the forearm bone, while ulna loops slope towards the inner ulna. Henry then divided his five classifications into sub-patterns, and he also devised a system for counting papillary lines such as Vucetich had done. These resulted in further sub-divisions.

As Peter Laurie puts it in his book *Scotland Yard*; 'To the layman, Henry's system appears to be one of the most obscure inventions of the human mind.' But Henry's native Bengal policemen soon mastered his technique, and over a short period of years secured remarkable successes with it. On 12 July 1897, the Governor General of India ordered anthropometry to be totally discontinued in the country, in favour of what Henry magnanimously insisted should be termed the Galton-Henry system of dactyloscopy. Twelve months later, Henry published his book *The Classification and Uses of Finger Prints*. It remains a standard police text book on the subject in every country in which the Galton-Henry system is used.

It was the Troup Committee, under the guidance of the then British Home Secretary, Herbert Henry Asquith, which first made a thorough investigation of the fingerprint system as far as Britain – and through its influence Europe in general – was concerned. In 1894 it reported among other things that:

The chance of two fingerprints being identical is less than one in sixty four thousand millions. It is wholly inconceivable that two persons should show an exact coincidence in the prints of two or three, let alone ten, fingers.

Three years later the Belper Committee reported to the Government that bertillonage should be discontinued and that the Galton-Henry system be adopted; Henry received a knighthood and, in 1901, became Assistant Commissioner of the Criminal Investigation Department of New Scotland Yard, setting up its first Fingerprint Branch the same year.

Rapidly, the Galton-Henry system spread to the law enforcement agencies of the United States; by 1903 prisoners arriving at Sing Sing and other jails in New York State were automatically fingerprinted; and the following year the St Louis Police Department, Missouri, set up a fingerprint department, blazing the trail for other national forces. Today, the South American countries and China are the only places to cling wholly to Vucetich's methods, although a combination of the Henry and Vucetich systems is used in France, Belgium, and Egypt; while the systems used in Germany and Italy are slight modifications of the Galton-Henry method. All are enhanced by the 'single print' system developed from the Galton-Henry system by Superintendent Harry Battley of Scotland Yard in the 1920s, so that today chance impressions of even a portion of a single fingerprint left at the scene of a crime can be rapidly identified.

Of the three early innovators in the field of criminal identification, only Sir Edward Henry received the recognition he deserved; both Vucetich and Bertillon were to die disappointed and frustrated men.

For Bertillon, who had worked so hard against the scorn of his Paris superiors to build up confidence in his system, only to have its flaws exposed not once but several times, the cup was particularly bitter. Two cases within as many years of each other cancelled out any lingering doubts that British and American criminologists might have had as to the infallibility of his system.

The first occurred in England in 1901, and not only showed the deficiences of bertillonage, but also made an important point about the nature of fingerprints.

Two waggish identical twins, Albert Ebenezer Fox and his brother Ebenezer Albert Fox, were arrested for poaching; only one was actually guilty according to the circumstantial evidence

– but which one ? The twins kept up a smug silence. The police tried bertillonage in an effort to distinguish between them; all 14 of their measurements were exactly identical. Then their fingerprints were taken and, of course the difference was spotted immediately. Ebenezer Albert was convicted, and when Assistant Commissioner Henry heard of the case he was as delighted as Albert Ebenezer, the twin who went free.

Two years later and several thousand miles away, a Negro named Will West was taken to Fort Leavenworth Prison, Kansas, after conviction. At the reception area he was measurep and his card, No. 3246, was made out and his photograph pasted onto it. The guard leafed through the filing system and suddenly bellowed with rage. He pulled out a card and waved it under the startled prisoner's nose.

'What the hell are you trying to pull ?' he yelled. 'According to this card you've been here for eight months. Who are you trying to fool ? Nice stunt you've figured out to get off work for a while.'

The prisoner looked at the second card. It was numbered 2626, but the measurements on it were identical with his, and the photograph which stared up at him seemed to be his own picture. Angrily the guard sent to the workrooms to find out why West was not at his post. But it was his turn for astonishment when word came back that he had not left the work area. So despite appearances, measurements, and even name, the Will West on card 3246 was not the Will West of card 2626.

Leavenworth's Warden McCloughty ordered the two men brought before him and checked the measurements personally. They tallied. Then he remembered the 'new-fangled' fingerprint system he had read about. Using a simple ink-pad and paper, he ordered the two men to press their prints onto the paper, and then examined them through a magnifying glass. The difference was immediately obvious. McCloughty is said to have yelled: 'This is the end of bertillonage!' The very next day he stopped anthropometry at Leavenworth, and ordered books and equipment on the Galton-Henry method.

Bertillon himself was involved in the sensational crime which finally broke confidence in his system as it stood in his native France. In 1911, the Mona Lisa was stolen from the Louvre by an incredibly daring but unhinged Italian named Vincenzo Perugia whose motive was to restore the painting to Italy where, he claimed, it rightfully belonged.

Despite public outcry and frenetic police activity, the crime remained unsolved for two years. Bertillon had been called to the Louvre in person, and in fact had found clear prints on the glass case of the painting – but he could not name their owner, because although he had taken to adding fingerprints to his records, he obstinately filed them as 'special marks'. When Perugia tried to sell the painting and was finally captured, it was discovered that not only had he been gaoled on several occasions before in Paris, but that Bertillon had taken both his measurements and his prints.

When the details reached the newspapers, Bertillon's popularity waned as quickly as it had begun. His illnesses increased, and his sight began to fail. Pernicious anaemia was diagnosed, and he died on 13 February 1914.

A few months before he died, Bertillon was visited by another man doomed to disappointment: Juan Vucetich. Vucetich had been in France and merely wanted to compliment Bertillon on his pioneering work. Bertillon, however, slammed the door in his face, crying: 'Sir, you have tried to do me great wrong!'

The incident depressed Vucetich, particularly as it was becoming clear that his own system had been overtaken by the Galton-Henry alternative, and was unlikely ever to find favour outside his native South America. And he was right; despite world-wide tours which he made to advertise his system, he died in misery on 28 July 1925. Thus the fight to bring criminal identification into the modern world was not without its heartbreak.

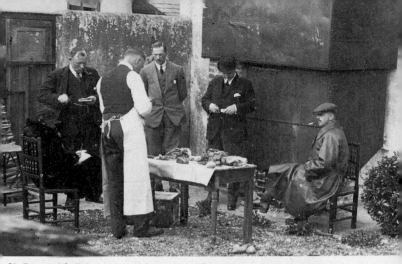

Sir Bernard Spilsbury at work in the case of the Eastbourne bungalow murder in 1924. Called in by the police, he discovered 42 pieces of human body (Syndication International)

Some of the case cards kept by Sir Bernard Spilsbury, with comprehensive details of his post-mortem examinations (from *Bernard Spilsbury: His Life and Cases* by D. G. Browne and T. Tullet)

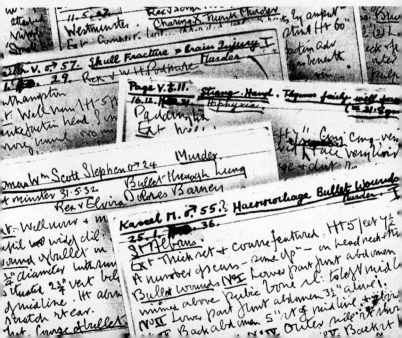

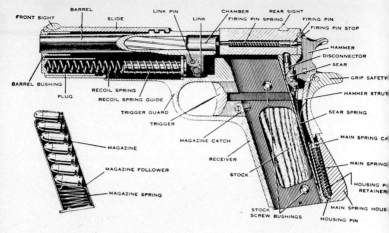

The working parts of the Colt .45 'automatic' pistol, showing clearly the rifling of the barrel, and the way in which a seven-round magazine fits into the pistol grip

A sheet of card prepared by the British Metropolitan Police forensic laboratory to show powder stains from a .32 Colt revolver at different distances (Metropolitan Police)

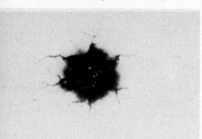

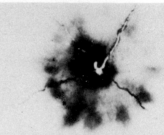

Bullet found in body | Bullet from suspect's gun | The two bullets compared

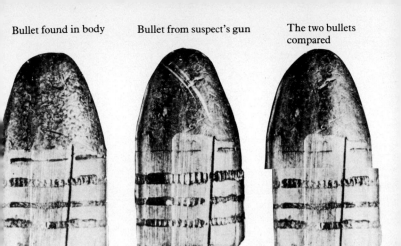

Matching the striations on a bullet found in the body of a murdered person with those on a bullet fired by the gun of a suspect (Radio Times Hulton Picture Library)

The fingerprint form used by the British police has recently been modified, but the majority of records are as the example shown here (Metropolitan Police)

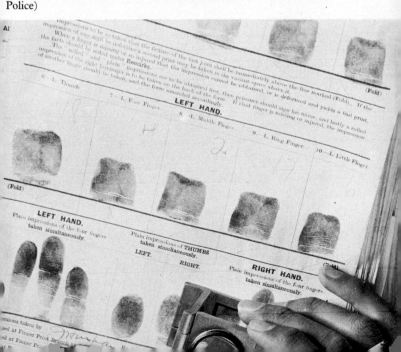

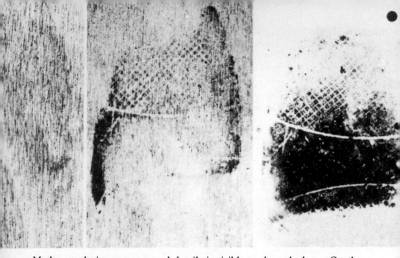

Modern techniques can reveal details invisible to the naked eye. On the left is a shoeprint made on a wood surface in which no detail is visible, but under infrared light (centre) more details are shown up, which compare closely with the iodine-developed paper print (right) taken from a suspect's shoe

A clear bruise-print from a boot on the forehead of an unfortunate victim (Metropolitan Police)

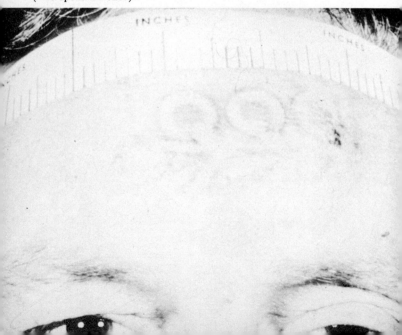

A broken knife found in a suspect's possession, fitted to the tip of the knife found in the victim's skull (Metropolitan Police)

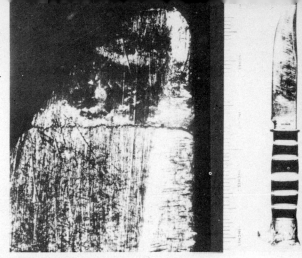

A human hair magnified 240 times (left) compared with a dog's hair (Ken Moreman)

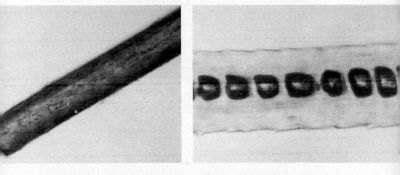

The shape of blood splashes at the scene indicates the direction and distance from which the blood was splashed. On the right, characteristic 'exclamation mark' splashes from an angle of 60 degrees and (left) from directly above (Metropolitan Police)

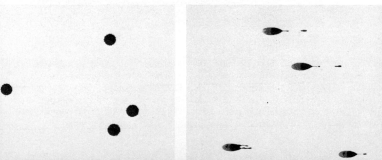

# INTERESTING SPEECH PATTERN

WE

YOU

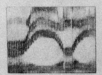

REALLY

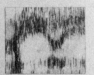

REALLY (WHISPERED)

## NUMBERS FREQUENTLY CONFUSED

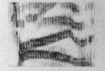

FIVE

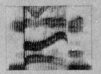

NINE

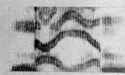

NIYAN

## WORDS THAT SOUND ALIKE LOOK ALIKE

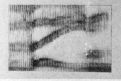

VEIN

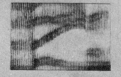

VANE

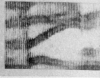

VAIN

One of the most exciting developments in forensic science in recent years has been the acceptance of 'voiceprints' in evidence. Much of the experimental work is due to L. G. Kersta of the Bell Telephone Company laboratories, who prepared the prints shown here. They show how similar word sounds produce similar speech patterns, strikingly exemplified in the voiceprints of the words 'vein', 'vane' and 'vain' (John Topham Picture Library)

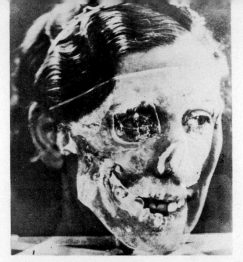

The human skull can survive for an enormous length of time unchanged, and can provide an unrivalled means of identification. This is the skull believed to have belonged to Mrs Ruxton. It fitted her photograph closely, particularly in the position of the eyes and the teeth (John Topham Picture Library)

Richard Speck, found guilty of the murder of eight student nurses in Chicago, 1966. The telltale tattoo which, with its inscription 'Born to Raise Hell', positively identified the killer can be seen on his right forearm (Popperfoto)

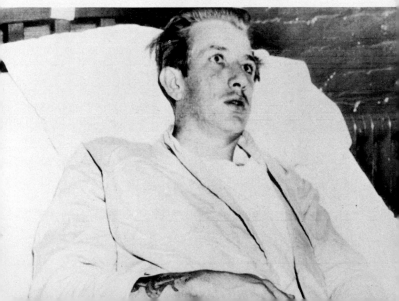

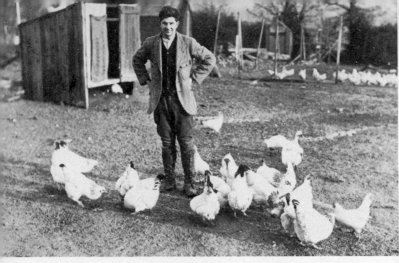

Thomas Thorne poses for press photographers near Crowborough. He stands on the spot where the body of Elsie Cameron was later found buried (Radio Times Hulton Picture Library)

Dr Crippen in the Old Bailey dock with his unwitting 'accomplice', Ethel le Neve, 1910

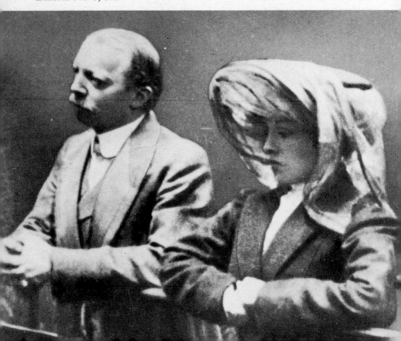

# Chapter Seven
# Finger of suspicion

The Moving Finger writes, and having writ
Moves on; nor all thy Piety and Wit
Shall lure it back to cancel half a line.

Edward Fitzgerald, *The Rubbaiyat of Omar Khayyam*

When the wonders of dactyloscopy became widespread public knowledge at the turn of the century, there was no shortage of enthusiastic churchmen ready to claim that the significance of fingerprints, like many other things, had been pointed out in the Bible. They quoted Job 37: 7. 'He sealeth up the hand of every man.'

Chief Superintendent Fred Cherrill, who was head of Scotland Yard's Fingerprint Department for over thirty years, was highly amused at this piece of special pleading. For his part, he liked to quote another passage from the Old Testament: II Kings 9: 34-37.

'See now this cursed woman, and bury her: for she is a king's daughter. And they went to bury her: but they found no more of her than the skull, and the feet, and the palms of her hands ... so that they shall not say, This is Jezebel.'

In the introduction to his book *The Finger Print System at Scotland Yard* Cherrill comments:

... those are the very remains by which a corpse might most surely be identified. If fingerprint identification was practised in the East in those days, one wonders whether Jehu would not have taken precautions to dispose of these tell-tale remains.

Certainly, any modern police force would expect to have little difficulty with Jezebel's remains as described, the techniques of identifying both criminals and their victims having progressed steadily since the days of Bertillon, Henry and Vucetich. It was Cherrill himself who did more than anyone else to improve upon the fingerprinting of both the living and the dead during his tenure of office, and though Peter Laurie, in his book *Scotland*

129

*Yard*, quotes a young fingerprint officer as saying 'What we want is four fingers, upside down in a bunch under the window sill. He has to be a housebreaker' – this is simply the ideal.

'One square centimetre of one finger contains enough detail to identify a man uniquely,' he goes on, 'but before two prints can be said in court to be the same, sixteen matching peculiarities must be found. Then big photographs are made for the jury with rings drawn round each one of the sixteen points, and lines to join the similarities.'

Forensic scientist Stuart Kind and his co-author Michael Overman, in their book *Science Against Crime*, mention several curious cases in which fingerprint experts seem to have surpassed themselves. In one case, a housebreaker wore surgical gloves while going to work, stripping them off and discarding them as he fled. Police turned the gloves inside out and were able to obtain clear prints from the insides of the gloves to secure a conviction.

In another case, scene-of-crime officers in the north of England found very odd looking prints on the smooth surfaces of a room which had been burgled. Further inquiries led them to a known criminal who happened to have a pair of pig-skin gloves in his possession. One original-thinking policeman took impressions from these gloves, and was able to show that they had made the marks in the burgled house. Confronted with the evidence the burglar confessed.

But perhaps the most remarkable case of all concerned a woman who had been attacked by an unknown man; she had successfully beaten off her assailant, and was taken to hospital to be treated for cuts and brusing of the face. While examining her lips, the doctor found a small fragment of skin wedged between two of her lower teeth, and removed it with tweezers. He noticed a pattern of ridges and realized that it was probably from her attacker's finger; the woman remembered biting the man. Examining it, police experts discovered that it bore part of the pattern of a fingertip whorl and made a print of it.

A few hours later, a police officer noticed a man with an injured finger and took him to the police station. The man claimed to have injured the finger at work, but his prints were taken. The print of his left middle finger showed that a piece of skin had been torn from the centre of the fingertip pattern, and the experts were quickly able to show that the portion of skin recovered from the woman's mouth matched the torn fingertip exactly.

Though unusual, none of these cases presented any special problems to the modern experts confronted with them for, using today's methods, fingerprints may be taken from almost any surface of contact, including certain fabrics and even human skin. Contrary to popular belief, a surprising number of real life criminals fail to wear gloves while committing their crimes, and, as has been seen, gloves by no means offer the complete protection that writers of fiction would have us believe.

Basically, fingerprint impressions come under three types: the latent print, the visible print, and the plastic, or moulded, print. Of these three the most frequent, and therefore most important to crime fighters, is the first variety.

Latent prints are formed by sweat from either the palms themselves or by unconscious contact between the fingers and the face or other parts of the body where the sebaceous glands are situated – the greasy parts of the skin. This means that though the criminal may scrub his hands clean and dry them thoroughly, if he then puts a hand to his face he is likely to leave a latent print, invisible to the naked eye, on anything he touches, particularly on such surfaces as glass or polished wood.

The second variety of fingerprint, the 'visible' kind, is perhaps the most dramatic and is thus a favourite of detective fiction writers; but it is in fact the rarest. Visible prints are formed by fingers stained with blood or ink or some other similar medium, and only the most incompetent or agitated criminal leaves them at the scene of the crime. The same thing goes for the third category, the plastic print, which is an impression made on a soft surface such as soap, cheese, or putty. So it is with the latent print that most criminal investigations are concerned.

The life of a latent print is variable and governed by several factors, but it is true to say that, made on a hard, protected surface and left untouched, it is almost permanent; latent prints have been found and developed from objects in ancient tombs.

In order to 'develop' a latent print, the fingerprint officer dusts very delicately over any likely surfaces at the scene of the crime, using a fine grained powder and a camel hair brush. The most common powder in use in the United States and Britain is 'grey' powder, a mixture of ground chalk and mercury, but 'white' powders, such as white lead powder made from basic lead carbonate, or French chalk, are used for dusting dark surfaces such as gun-metal or tinted wine bottles. Conversely, darker agents such as carbon black are used to develop prints on light paintwork or china.

Most experienced scene-of-crime officers have their own preferences and mix powders to suit their own needs, just as different officers will handle the dusting brush in slightly different ways, though the actual skill involved in dusting is likely to disappear within the next decade or so. An American forensic scientist, Herbert L. Macdonnell, developed a magnetic 'brush' in the 'sixties in which the 'bristles' are actually made up of magnetic fingerprint powder held in a magnetic field; this device is designed to bestow lightness of touch on even the most heavy handed operator. Aerosol spraying has also been proposed.

The Macdonnell brush has proved particularly useful where fluorescent powder has to be used, in cases where the surface to be dusted is multi-coloured or presents other difficulties. Until now the use of fluorescent powder has required a very delicate touch indeed; after dusting, the print is exposed to ultraviolet light, which shows it up in order that it can be photographed. If a fraction too much powder is used, the print appears as an oval blob, and is useless. The use of the magnetic brush has effectively removed the possibility of prints being destroyed in such a way.

Prints on paper need special treatment, though again the techniques are straightforward enough. Latent prints on high-gloss cardboard or even shiny paper can be dusted in the ordinary way, but the operator has to be very quick before the sweat and grease forming the print sink into the porous surface. Normally where paper is concerned, the iodine fuming process is brought into play.

This process will show up all kinds of marks on paper, even some forms of secret writing. The paper to be examined is placed, face downward, over a straight-sided glass tray, about half an inch above some well-distributed iodine crystals. The iodine will quite rapidly sublime at room temperature, and within five minutes will reveal any prints on the paper. The prints must be photographed rapidly, as the iodine will in turn evaporate quite soon from the paper surface.

A rather more modern method of developing prints from paper or other porous materials involves the use of the reagent ninhydrin. The surface is sprayed with aerosol containing a solution of ninhydrin in acetone; as the acetone evaporates the surface is gently heated and the latent prints show up reddish-blue, due to the reaction of amino acids in the prints with the ninhydrin. The two major drawbacks to the widespread use of this technique are that the amino acid content of sweat varies from person to person, in some cases being too weak to show, and that acetone dissolves certain inks and so has to be used with extreme care on printed papers such as documents.

Yet another technique for developing latent prints, not only on paper but also in finely woven cloth, involves the use of silver nitrate solution, which reacts with the sodium chloride – ordinary salt – which forms up to one third of the content of human sweat. In this case, the paper or cloth is either brushed with or dipped in the silver nitrate solution, and the solution reacts with the salt present to form sodium nitrate and silver chloride. Silver chloride is both indissoluble in water and sensitive to light, so that when the object under examination is rinsed in distilled water, the sodium nitrate is washed off, leaving in effect a photograph of any latent prints outlined in silver chloride.

There are various other methods, differing only in the chemicals used, for obtaining fingerprints from other surfaces; the prints of a sex murderer may sometimes be developed on the dead body of his victim by treating the smoother areas of the body – the back or breasts, for instance – with a solution of benzidine, alcohol, and hydrogen peroxide. Certain metals are best treated with fine copper powder, while materials such as satin or silk are dusted with calcium sulphide. In every case, the object is to develop a print clear enough to photograph, and over the years criminal photography has developed to keep pace with modern needs. Light filters, oblique lighting, and filtered ultraviolet light are all used to various ends, and police technicians have developed camera and lens attachments to deal with almost every contingency which may arise.

Despite all those sophisticated techniques, not every crime yields up convenient fingerprints to its investigators, largely because prints can be destroyed, either accidentally or otherwise. Real life policemen often find the activities of their television counterparts risible in the extreme.

'For instance,' said a Scotland Yard scene-of-crime man, 'I'm always amused when the telly cop goes to extraordinary lengths to dust a door handle and comes up triumphant. In fact it is almost impossible to turn a handle or knob and leave a clear print on it; the hand always slides fractionally, so that the print is smeared and useless.'

The common fictional habit of wrapping suspect objects in handkerchiefs is similarly ridiculous, again because the lightest touch – whether of clean linen or clumsy hands – can spoil a print.

'And when I see Kojak sticking a pencil into a barrel of a suspect gun to pick it up I come out in a cold sweat,' said the Yard man. 'The ballistics people examine the inside of a gun barrel as minutely as we check out fingerprints; a pencil shoved up it in such a way could ruin valuable evidence.'

The standard procedure for removing a revolver or automatic hand gun from the scene of a crime is either to insert wire through the lanyard eye in the gun butt, if the model has one, or to grip the sides of the trigger guard with a pair of pliers. In any case, ideally, investigating officers are instructed to keep their hands firmly in their pockets and touch nothing at the scene of the crime until the experts arrive – unless of course they need to check that a suspected murder victim is actually dead.

In all cases of death by violence, the finger, palm (and, if appropriate, sole) prints of the dead body are taken as a matter of routine, and this presents special and sometimes unpleasant problems. The prints are needed for three main reasons: to eliminate from the investigation any prints left at the scene by the victim, to help with identification by comparison with latent prints made by the victim during life, and to prove or disprove any contention leading up to the cause of death.

In this field of dactyloscopy as in others, Chief Superintendent Cherrill was a pioneer, and his methods are still used throughout the world. In his textbook on fingerprint methods, he details procedures for toughening up the skin of decomposing corpses using formaldehyde and alum, unwrinkling dead skin by injecting wax with a hypodermic, and softening hard skin by simmering the finger in a saline solution or soaking it in caustic potash – a difficult operation to judge with accuracy.

One of the most spectacularly macabre processes evolved by Cherrill, in conjunction with his friend and colleague Sir Bernard Spilsbury, involved the peeling off of the whole skin of a dead hand as if it were a tight-fitting glove. This grisly operation was made much easier if the body was macerated – long immersed in water either through drowning or in an attempt to get rid of the corpse – for the skin of such bodies, along with the nails, sloughs off within two to four weeks of immersion.

One of Cherrill's triumphs in this direction is detailed by Douglas Browne and E. V. Tullett in their biography of Spilsbury. In 1938 the legless body of a woman was found rolling in the surf off a beach in Cornwall. Most of the flesh was gone, and the scarification of the sand had worn and polished the protruding bones. When he examined the body Cherrill found that the fingerprint ridges too had been worn away as smoothly as if filed with an emery board. Nevertheless: 'Cherrill performed the extremely delicate task of peeling off the rotting skin, revealing on the underside the pattern of ridges, loops and whorls reversed. Faint though these were, he obtained recognisable prints.'

In this case, unfortunately, Cherrill's efforts came to naught. Spilsbury's post-mortem and the subsequent police inquiries showed that the body was almost certainly that of a woman who had committed suicide by jumping overboard from a ship. Accordingly, Cherrill set out for the woman's home in the north of England.

His journey served only to illustrate the least pleasing side of human nature. The relatives had forestalled him. One of them had observed that if they claimed to identify the body it would mean the expense of a funeral, but there was more to it than that – there was an insurance policy with a suicide clause – and when Cherrill examined the room where he hoped to compare his fingerprints he found that every inch of the floors and walls, the doors, cupboards, and furniture, had been scrubbed and polished clean.

Eleven years later, when the headless and legless torso of a man was found in the Essex marshes, Cherrill had better luck. He peeled the hands, treated the skin with glycerine, and was able to identify the corpse as that of Stanley Setty, a shady car dealer with a criminal record. As a result a man named Donald Hume was quickly arrested and tried for Setty's killing. Hume escaped the death penalty on a technicality, served a sentence for being an accessory to murder, and then, on release, confessed that he had stabbed Setty, cut up his body to avoid identification, and scattered the pieces from a light airplane. In 1959, ten years after the Setty slaying, Hume killed again, this time a Zurich taxi driver, and was sentenced to life imprisonment.

During the course of his career, Cherrill saw several attempts, on the part of criminals, to destroy or mutilate their own fingerprints in an attempt to evade conviction; he came to the conclusion that such attempts were futile. Unless the flesh of the fingertips is removed down to and beneath the dermal layer of skin – the lowermost – the prints eventually grow again into their original pattern. And were such an operation possible, the very presence of massive scarring would alert the police.

Nevertheless, several determined efforts were made in the comparatively early days of fingerprinting to eliminate fingertip marks, principally by American mobsters. The first such case came to light in January 1934 when three FBI agents gunned down a Chicago gangster named 'Pretty Jack' Klutas. Klutas was a cut above his contemporaries in intelligence; a graduate of the University of Illinois, he specialized in kidnapping and blackmailing fellow members of the underworld in the certain knowledge that they would not appeal to the police for help.

When FBI men attempted to take his fingerprints for identification, they found, to their astonishment, that his fingertips were smooth. J. Edgar Hoover himself was told of the alarming discovery, and ordered skin specialists from Northwestern University to examine the dead man's hands. To the relief of Hoover – and the FBI's fingerprint department – it was found that Klutas had undergone an operation to remove the upper layers of skin from his fingers, but that his old papillary ridges were already beginning to show on the new skin.

Five months later, two members of the notorious 'Ma Barker' gang decided to follow Klutas's lead. Al Karpis and Freddie Barker were high on the list of FBI priorities and, in hiding, they not only dyed their hair and took to wearing dark glasses but contacted a drunken abortionist named Dr Joseph P. Moran, whose 'practice' consisted largely of patching up wounded mobsters. Moran visited the Barker hideout and performed an operation to remove the flesh from the two mens' fingertips; he bungled it so badly that, despite heavy morphine sedation, Karpis and Barker screamed with pain for days. At the end of four weeks their bandages were removed only for them to discover that their papillary ridges were already showing through the scar tissue again. The furious Karpis paid Dr Moran by taking him out in a boat into Lake Michigan and dumping him over the side.

At exactly the same time as the Karpis-Barker operations were taking place, John Dillinger, dubbed by Hoover 'Public Enemy Number 1', was also undergoing an operation, this time for plastic surgery. Dillinger's doctors were vastly more competent than the unfortunate Moran; they were the German Dr Wilhelm Loeser, an expert in facial surgery, and his assistant Dr Harold Cassedy. Loeser and Cassedy operated on Dillinger's face, but the gangster was dissatisfied with the results. He asked Loeser to operate on his fingerprints too, to make the disguise a little more complete. Unlike Moran, Loeser decided to treat the fingertips with acid, and this time he seemed to be successful. But the results were only temporary. When Dillinger was killed by FBI agents outside the Biograph Cinema, Chicago, on 22 July 1934, the tell-tale lines were showing once more.

The last major attempt to disguise human fingerprints by surgery took place in May 1941, at the home of a New Jersey doctor named Leopold Brandenburg – again a physician who had run foul of the law. His patient was a car thief and armed robber named Robert J. Philipps, alias 'Roscoe' Pitts. Brandenburg had studied previous efforts at fingertip disguise, and tried a new approach; he grafted skin from Philipps' chest onto the fingers in a operation which took almost a month to complete. In October of the same year, Philipps was arrested in Austin, Texas, for not carrying a draft card. The astonishment of officials at his apparent lack of prints soon turned to determination as they searched files and dossiers on known criminals in an effort to establish his real identity. Finally they came up with the record they needed: Philipps had been arrested for car theft in Virginia some years before, and though Brandenburg had done a good job of removing the prints from the top phalange of his fingers, prints of the second phalange tallied with those on the Virginia file. His identity was proved, he had failed to outsmart the FBI.

The fact that his own fingerprints are liabilities which are always with him is accepted by the average professional criminal today; if he leaves his 'marks' at the scene of a crime, he has only himself to blame. From time to time, however, a villain may try another approach in an attempt to escape punishment, and claim that his fingerprints have been 'rigged' either by the police or a criminal rival in order to frame him.

In fact, the only way to achieve this would be by obtaining a genuine print on a moveable object and leaving the object at the scene of the crime. It is impossible to 'forge' a print in such a way as to fool a fingerprint expert.

Of course, a skilled craftsman could make a rubber copy of a human fingerprint without a great deal of difficulty, but the impression of such an artificial 'stamp' would not stand up to laboratory investigation, and would in fact be spotted fairly quickly by an ordinary police technician. The processes which deposit human sweat to make up a normal latent print cannot be reproduced artificially, but there are two even simpler objections. The use of a magnifying glass to examine any artificially impressed print would show up the ridges as being unnatural, and would also reveal the absence of pore mouths. Finally, a print made by a rubber stamp device cannot be 'lifted', as an ordinary latent print can, on a strip of clear Sellotape.

There is an American case which shows up the difficulty of fingerprint faking. A criminal seeking revenge on a former colleague obtained one of his fingerprints and had it reproduced in rubber stamp form; he then robbed a garage and left rubber 'prints' at four carefully chosen sites. When the police found them they were struck immediately by the fact that all four prints began and ended at specific ridges; and measurement showed their width and breadth to be identical to the last millimetre. The flexibility of human skin would, of course, rule out such a series of coincidences in the case of a real print.

Nevertheless, there have been rare cases of unscrupulous police officers 'bending' fingerprint evidence to suit their own ends; in one of the most dramatic examples the false testimony of a fingerprint officer came within an ace of sending Count Marie Alfred Fouquereau de Marigny to the gallows.

'Freddy' de Marigny was a wealthy playboy who lived near Nassau, in the Bahamas, with his heiress-bride, the beautiful eighteen-year-old Nancy Oakes. Nancy's father, Sir Harry Oakes, was a millionaire mine owner who was also a social climber; born in Maine in 1874, he had made his money as a prospector in the Klondike and had later moved to the Bahamas, where he became a British citizen. Through generous gifts to charity he gained a knighthood in 1939. In 1942 de Marigny ran off to New York with Nancy and married her there; Oakes was furious and the rift was never quite healed, particularly as the rich knight liked people to be dependent upon him, and de Marigny, with his own money, needed nothing from Sir Harry.

What particularly annoyed Oakes, and the rest of the white socialites of the Bahamas, was de Marigny's arrogant attitude to the Governor, formerly King Edward VIII of England, now Duke of Windsor, and his wife, the former Mrs Wallace Simpson. On several public occasions the elegant de Marigny had cut them dead.

All this dissension was remembered when, in the first week of July 1943, Sir Harry Oakes was found murdered in the master bedroom of his home at Westbourne, near Nassau. It was a particularly horrific scene; Sir Harry's head had been battered in, and his blood splashed across the bed, the walls, and the furniture. And gasolene had been poured on his naked body and ignited, searing his face and genitals.

After the first investigation by the Nassau police, the Duke of Windsor stepped in. Despite suggestions that he use the services of either the FBI or Scotland Yard, he sent for Captain Edward Melchen of the Miami police, who brought with him Captain James O. Barker, of the Miami Crime Laboratory; both officers had previously been attached to the Duke in an official capacity.

The two policemen quickly found a number of circumstantial pointers which indicated that de Marigny could have committed the crime, but only one truly damning piece of evidence; on a Chinese screen in the dead man's room was, they alleged, the clear fingerprint of the little finger, right hand, of de Marigny.

Nancy Oakes did not believe for a moment that her husband would have killed her father, and called in the celebrated New York private investigator Raymond Campbell Schindler. Schindler, whose asthmatically plump frame belied a brilliant grasp of criminology, flew out to the Bahamas and, after investigating the circumstances of Oakes's death, had to agree with Nancy. Her husband could have killed his father-in-law, but taking everything into consideration the investigator felt it unlikely. The only point that worried him was the fingerprint.

But Schindler soon found that many different fingerprints had been left in Sir Harry's room after his death, largely due to the fact that the police had allowed visitors and servants to wander in and handle ornaments and fittings. Captain Barker, the so-called fingerprint expert, had ruined several whole-hand prints in blood by dusting them before they had dried, and the thought occurred to Schindler that such incompetence in a man of Barker's reputation could only be deliberate.

The 'evidence' of the fingerprint made him even more suspicious. To begin with it had been 'lifted' from the screen on which it was said to have been deposited with a piece of clear tape, before being photographed – a procedure normally used only when the object on which the print appears is immovable. The Chinese screen was light enough to lift with one hand.

Nor had Barker kept to the standard police procedure of taking a photograph of the developed print *in situ*. When asked why, he answered feebly that his camera was broken.

Schindler now called in one of the leading fingerprint experts in the world, Maurice O'Neill of New Orleans. O'Neill was intrigued by the 'lifted' print: it had a background of circles under it. Over a period of weeks, Schindler and O'Neill examined every single print on the surface of the screen, lifted them all, and subjected them to rigorous scrutiny. None of them bore the circular marks which showed on the de Marigny print. Most curious of all was the fact that when they examined the exact spot from which Barker claimed he had lifted his print no mark, not even a smudged one, existed. The only possible explanation was that Barker had rigged the evidence to convict de Marigny.

When Schindler presented the evidence to two able lawyers hired on behalf of de Marigny, the Supreme Court of the Bahamas had no alternative but to clear the accused man. Barker was ruined, became addicted to drugs and, ten years later, was shot by his own son. The episode served to highlight the necessity to consider fingerprint evidence very carefully. In any case, the true murderer was never brought to justice.

Five years after de Marigny's acquittal a new development in the use of fingerprinting by the forces of law and order posed another question which has been debated ever since. On the night of 14 May 1948, a four-year-old girl named June Anne Devaney disappeared from her bed in the children's ward of Queen's Park Hospital, Blackburn, in the north of England. At 11 pm a night nurse had noticed that the child was sleeping soundly; three quarters of an hour later she found a window open and June's bed empty. Hurriedly, the nurse searched the toilet area and found that empty too, but despite her rising panic she noticed something; there were footmarks on the freshly polished ward floor leading to and from June Devaney's bed, and by the bed was a large bottle of distilled water which must, the nurse realized, have been moved from a trolley during her absence from the room.

The nurse called the police immediately, and at three o'clock in the morning the child's body was found by the hospital boundary. She had been sexually molested, and her head battered against the wall.

Chief Inspector Campbell of the Lancashire Police fingerprint department made a preliminary examination of the ward and found clear prints on the bottle. Scotland Yard was contacted, and the same morning Chief Inspector John Capstick arrived with Murder Squad detectives. A further examination of the scene showed that the footprints on the waxed floor had been made by a man in stockinged feet, and Capstick concluded that he had picked up the heavy bottle for possible use as a weapon.

For four days, Chief Inspector Campbell checked the prints on the bottle with those of anyone who might have entered the ward, even weeks before; doctors, nurses, children, parents, porters, cleaners, visitors – all were checked. Gradually all were eliminated and Campbell surmised that the prints on the bottle must be those of the murderer. With public outcry growing, the prints were sent to every police fingerprint department in Britain and several abroad. All efforts proved fruitless. Then Campbell made a unique and, to the police, potentially outrageous suggestion: that the prints of all male inhabitants of Blackburn over the age of sixteen be taken for comparison.

The Mayor of Blackburn made the request public – for, of course, its success depended entirely on voluntary contributions of prints. On behalf of the Chief Constable he promised that all prints would be destroyed after the operation; that none would be used for checking against those of men wanted for other, lesser crimes; and finally that the prints would be taken on a door-to-door basis, so that no-one need be seen going to a police station.

There were 110,000 people resident in Blackburn at the time. Chief Inspector Campbell reckoned that the survey would need 50,000 fingerprint sheets. Nevertheless he began his mammoth task of collecting and checking, and by early August 45,000 sets of prints were on file. Unfortunately, none tallied. Then a ration card officer – rationing of certain goods continued in Britain for several years after World War II – suggested checking the males on the latest ration card list. When this was done it was discovered that almost eight hundred had yet to give their prints to the police. On 11 August, one of the missing men called upon was 22-year-old Peter Griffiths, who lived with his mother and was said to be a 'decent young man' by the neighbours. He had also spent long spells in the Queen's Park Hospital as a child, and knew the layout and routine of the place. His prints were those on the bottle; he confessed to the murder.

The success of Chief Inspector Campbell's mass fingerprinting idea sparked a controversy not only in Britain but abroad: if national registration of prints – as suggested by Juan Vucetich over sixty years previously – had been in force, June Devaney's murderer would have been caught within hours. The killer might even have been deterred from his crime, knowing that his prints were already in police hands.

J. Edgar Hoover had long advocated the idea in America. In 1956, figures showed that of the 140,000,000 fingerprints on the files of the government bureaux, over 112,000,000 were those of respectable citizens who had never been in trouble with the law, and whose prints were there for a variety of other reasons. These records have proved enormously valuable in identifying the victims of accidents and disasters, as well as in eliminating their owners from implication in crime. And suppose cheques, for instance, were printed on the 'clean print' paper now used by most police forces – which takes fingerprints without the mess of ink and pad: the possibility of fraud, if the banks had their own print files, and the cheque owner made his mark upon each cheque issued, would be tremendously reduced.

Unfortunately, public opinion has so far resisted the idea of a national fingerprint file for everyone, criminal and innocent alike; to the democratic mind the concept smacks of 'police state' tactics. And though voluntary mass fingerprintings like that at Blackburn have taken place successfully since it seems that it will be a long time before Juan Vucetich's wider idea is brought into practice, in the Western world at least.

# Chapter Eight
# In tooth and claw

... and we ourselves compell'd
Even to the teeth and forehead of our faults
To give in evidence.

Shakespeare, *Hamlet*, Act III Scene 2

Chief Superintendent Cherrill implied in his comment on the biblical description of Jezebel's remains that human skulls and feet come second only to the hands in providing the criminologist with a rich source of information. In fact some forensic odontologists – dental experts – would go further: dental records are likely to exist of any work done on human teeth, and teeth are among the most indestructible parts of the body, infinitely more durable than the skin of the hands. Professor Keith Simpson wrote in the British *Medico-Legal Review* in 1951: '. . . dental data, it is now realised, has come to provide detail of a kind comparable with the infinitesimal detail that was previously thought likely to be provided only by fingerprints.'

But if a skull with teeth gives an investigator a great deal go on, a pair of feet – or even a pair of well-worn shoes or a set of clear footprints – can tell the astute observer a considerable amount about the owner. Age, illness, profession and even sex can be reflected in the way a person walks, and in certain conditions the weight of an individual can be assessed from the relative depth of his footprints left in clay or other soft ground.

A cast taken from the indentation of a foot – or a tyre tread or similar object – in a plastic substance such as earth is called a 'moulage' from the French for 'casting' and one of the first recorded instances of such a cast being taken occurs in the memoirs of the great French detective Francois Vidocq. Investigating the attempted murder of a butcher near Paris, Vidocq visited the scene of the crime and found several clear footprints, a button with a scrap of cloth attached, and a torn piece of paper. He took a plaster cast of the footprints and was able to match the impression with the distinctive boot of a suspect; this and the other clues secured him a conviction. From that time – the second decade of the nineteenth century – the casting of footprints became established practice with the police forces of Europe.

Though relatively stiff substances such as mud or clay provide the best moulds for footprints, other media such as dust or even sand can provide clues to those who know how to look. Professor Sydney Smith recorded one such case remarkable, as he puts it, 'for the way in which two sciences, one very ancient and the other very modern, led to exactly the same conclusion'.

In the 1920s, while Smith was serving as medico-legal adviser to the Egyptian government, the body of a postman was found on the fringe of the desert outside Cairo. The man had been in the habit of walking between two villages some miles apart. He had been shot through the head, and though no trace of the bullet was found, Smith concluded that the wound had been made by a high velocity weapon such as a .303 rifle. Unfortunately that was as far as he could go: the surrounding dust and sand bore no apparent marks, and police inquiries failed to turn up any sign of a motive, much less a suspect.

At this point Russel Pasha, Commandant of the Cairo City Police, enlisted the aid of Bedouin trackers, taught from infancy to identify the tracks of their family and cattle in the seemingly featureless desert sand. 'They could without difficulty spot the tracks of different persons they knew,' wrote Smith, 'and could tell whether a person or animal was running or walking, whether loaded or free, and so on.'

In this instance, the Bedouin found sandal prints – totally invisible to the police – which led to the body from a spot about forty yards away where, they said, someone had knelt. A few yards from this spot the trackers found an empty .303 rifle cartridge.

After killing his victim and examining the body, the marksman had apparently taken off his sandals and had run barefoot towards an earth track; the Bedouin followed the footprints along this road, which also bore the marks of a motor car and four persons wearing boots, until they came to a fort where six members of the Camel Corps were encamped. Here the trail ended.

The next day the six Camel Corps soldiers and a number of other men were ordered to run barefoot across a prepared stretch of sand. The Bedouin immediately picked out the tracks identical to the ones they had followed from the murder site. The test was repeated twice more, and each time the suspect tracks were identified without difficulty. On the fourth occasion the suspect was excluded from the test and the Bedouin spotted the omission at once.

The police were now certain that they had their man, but the Cairo courts were prejudiced against using the unsupported evidence of Bedouin. Accordingly, Smith obtained samples of cartridges cases fired not only from the rifles of the six Camel Corps members but also from every other .303 rifle in the vicinity – a total of 53. Each was examined under Smith's home-made comparison microscope alongside the cartridge recovered from the scene of the crime; from the marks of the firing pin, the breech block, and the bolt he found it easy to identify the murder weapon – which belonged to the soldier whose footprints had been identified by the trackers. Faced with the evidence the soldier confessed; the postman had been having an illicit affair with his sister, and the soldier had killed him to avenge the family honour.

Even the most modern police techniques cannot match the natural ability of such men as the Bedouin, though science has gone a long way to conquering the difficulties of taking moulages from such substances as fine dust and even snow, and of lifting impressions from sharply sloping surfaces.

The normal, horizontal moulage is taken with plaster of Paris poured into a casting trough placed around the indentation; as plaster dries it swells slightly, showing up the finest details on the finished cast. Obviously, the weight of the plaster destroys impressions left in soft substances, and in these cases the print is sprayed with an aerosol containing cellulose acetate dissolved in acetone. When the acetone vaporizes, a fine skin of acetate is left in the mould, which is then used as the basis for a conventional cast.

To take prints from a sloping surface a substance known as silastomer is used. Silastomer is a silicone derivative which comes in liquid or paste form and is mixed with a hardener immediately prior to use. It solidifies within moments, and it has the added advantage of being non-adhesive, so that it can be lifted out without damaging the surface on which it is used.

As every detective knows, a criminal who might be meticulous in not leaving fingerprints is often very careless about his feet. Often he will kick in a door, running the risk – particularly if he is wearing rubber shoes – of leaving a dusty imprint on the painted surface. Similarly he may use his feet for leverage in moving a heavy object such as a safe into a more convenient position. Wherever such marks are found at the scene of a crime the tell-tale traces must be photographed and filed. Such items of apparently trivial evidence eventually helped to link a whole series of crimes, with the subsequent recovery of thousands of dollars' worth of goods.

The spate of robberies apparently began in the spring of 1945, when a thief broke into several houses in a New York State township. He left only one clue – the prints of the middle and ring finger of his right hand on a wine bottle. Unfortunately the prints were not on file, but the police photographed them. In November of the same year another break-in occurred in the town, and this time the intruder left behind the prints of his index and middle right fingers – the middle finger print matched the previous one, indicating that the same man was responsible. He also left a piece of ragged cloth, apparently part of a bed-spread.

A year passed before the thief struck again. This time there were no prints, but the impression of an unusual overshoe was found in the garden of one of the houses concerned; police took a cast and added it to their growing file. In August 1947, after a robbery in a neighbouring county, the impression of an equally unusual sneaker was discovered; it too, was cast and filed. A few days later the same sneaker print turned up after a store robbery; shortly after that it appeared again at the scene of yet another burglary, and this time it was accompanied by finger-prints. They tallied with the ones taken from the 1945 crime sites, and showed the police that the same man was involved in the whole series of thefts.

In November 1947 came the breakthrough. After a robbery at a gas station in Seneca Falls, New York, local police were given the registration number of a car which had been parked nearby. They traced the owner and searched his home. There they found not only stolen goods but a torn bedspread which exactly matched the piece of cloth found in November 1945. The householder confessed his part in the crimes, and implicated his uncle, who lived nearby. At the uncle's house, police found a pair of sneakers and a pair of overshoes which matched the impressions already on file; they also discovered that the uncle's prints fitted those of the culprit. Eventually the uncle and nephew confessed to over fifty unsolved burglaries, dating back over several years, and led the police to the goods they had stolen.

Sneakers, baseball boots and other canvas-and-rubber shoes tend to be among the favourite working footwear of such criminals as cat burglars because of their lightness and non-slip qualities. Unfortunately for their users they have drawbacks, too. Canvas is easily snagged, leaving fibres at the scene of the crime, and it also marks easily, giving investigators the opportunity of comparing stains on the shoe with substances on the entered premises. A minor classic of investigation along these lines took place in pre-war Edinburgh.

In October 1937 a draper's shop in the city was broken into and a small amount of goods and cash stolen. On a cash box in the shop was the left thumb print of a known housebreaker named Coogan, along with other blurred prints on a bottle. The police arrested Coogan at his home, and found him in the company of another notorious burglar from Glasgow. There was reason to believe that the Glasgow man had been implicated in the shop break-in, but the prints of both men – Coogan's from the cash box, his companion's from the bottle – yielded only nine points of resemblance, whereas sixteen are required for positive evidence of identification in court.

None of the stolen goods was found at Coogan's home, but the police removed a pair of grey cotton-and-rubber sneakers, which Coogan claimed were his. At the laboratory, scientists found that the instep of each shoe was deeply marked with patches of rust about four inches in diameter, flecked with what appeared to be black paint. Both the rubber and the cotton had been worn by friction.

An examination of a drain-pipe running up the side of the draper's shop revealed fibres of grey cotton and minute particles of rubber which matched the shoes; similarly, the rust and paint on the shoes tallied with that found on the pipe and, to clinch matters, strands of blue and red fibre clinging to the soles of the shoes were proved to come from a carpet in the shop. Coogan was convicted and sentenced to a term of imprisonment. Ironically, in an attempt to help his friend, the Glasgow burglar swore that the shoes were his; on his sworn statement and the evidence of the blurred fingerprints on the bottle he too was convicted and jailed.

As an interesting postscript, Coogan was killed in a fall shortly after his release, and on examination by the police pathologist his big toes proved to be almost prehensile, with thick pads of skin – the result of years of drain-pipe climbing.

Today, the taking of gelatin-glycerine casts from the inside of footwear is a commonplace of forensic science; like several other techniques the process appears to have been pioneered by Professor Sir Sydney Smith – again in Scotland in 1937.

In the autumn of that year, two strongly similar break-ins occurred in the town of Falkirk. In both cases a pair of shoes had been left behind, placed neatly by the drain-pipe which had apparently given access to the premises. On 28 November a third break-in took place, and this time the intruder was caught in his stockinged feet; a pair of boots, which he admitted were his, stood beside the drain-pipe. He denied any knowledge of the previous two crimes, however, and the police handed over all three pairs of footwear to Sir Sydney Smith for investigation.

Smith found that all three bore identical signs of wear. The right upper bulged over the base of the big toe, and the marks of the laces were more pronounced in the right foot than in the left; again, the right sole was worn thin, while the left one was almost unmarked. What markings there were on the left sole

149

were confined to the area of the toe, and formed a circular pattern. From this, Smith deduced that the wearer had suffered a deformity of the left foot, which tended to swivel while bearing weight.

At this point he injected the shoes with the gelatin-glycerine mixture, and produced casts of the feet themselves, and these told a very individual story. Smith pronounced – he had not so far seen the suspect – that the owner of the shoes had a deformity of the left leg and foot, both short and withered, which was characteristic of the results of infantile paralysis. He had walked with a limp, characterized by a swinging outward of the left big toe, and a dragging of the toe along the ground as he moved forward; he also suffered from curvature of the spine due to the pelvis being dipped to the affected side, and he was probably short in stature.

Professor Smith proved to be correct on all points, and the suspect was convicted of all three robberies. Smith's methods have been repeated with equal accuracy by criminal investigators all over the world in the forty-five years since then.

If feet – and their shoes – can be made to yield what amounts to a *portrait parlé* of their owners, then logically a human skull must be even more helpful to the forensic scientist. Anatomists have for years been able to tell the sex and race of a skull and the approximate age at death of the individual to whom it belonged, but it was not until the beginning of the present century that medico-legal experts began to consider the possibility of reconstructing the features of a dead man on to the facial bones.

The first attempt at such a reconstruction took place in New York in 1916, and apparently was a striking success. On 12 September a skeleton was found in a Brooklyn cellar. It was removed for examination to the mortuary, where measurements indicated it to be Italian; a scrap of hair clinging to the cranium was dark brown in colour, and using these facts as a basis police surgeons decided to try to rebuild the features. Rolled up newspapers formed the neck, brown eyes were fitted into the eye sockets, and the whole was covered with tinted plasticine, which was finished by a professional sculptor. The head was then put on display – with immediate success. Several Italians in the area named the dead man as one Domenico La Rosa, who had vanished some time previously, and all of them claimed that, apart from La Rosa's fuller cheeks, the image was exact; one relative even tried to part the lips to see if La Rosa's two gold teeth were still intact, a corroborative detail which the police had already noted.

But if the La Rosa case was a milestone in criminological history, most serious students of facial reconstruction agree that it was also something of a fortunate accident that the likeness, in this first case, was so exact. The technique of such reconstruction is beset by many problems, and it was not until almost two decades after the La Rosa affair that they were finally overcome, largely through the dedication, amounting to almost an obsession, of one man.

When he died in July 1970, Professor Mikhail Gerasimov was world famous not only in the field of palaeontology – his own discipline – but also in that of forensic medicine, for it was through his efforts that Russia came to the fore in the facial reconstruction branch of criminal science. As far back as 1950 Professor Gerasimov had been instrumental in the setting up of the Laboratory for Plastic Reconstruction, which forms part of the Ethnographical Institute of the USSR Academy of Sciences; since then the laboratory has assisted Russian investigators in the solving of hundreds of crimes.

Gerasimov was born in St Petersburg – later Leningrad – in 1907 and took a precocious interest in archaeology and palaeontology. As early as 1920, when he was 13, he had become a part-time student at the University of Irkutsk, in Siberia, attending lectures in archaeology, ethnography, zoology and medicine. He was also fortunate in gaining the patronage of Professor A. D. Grigoriev, holder of the chair of forensic science, who encouraged the youthful Gerasimov in his interest in the morphology of the human skull.

The task which faced Gerasimov was a complex one; firstly, he had to establish some form of set measurement from those parts of the skull which remained more or less constant – where, that is, the flesh lay thinnest on the bone. Then, much more difficult, he had to discover a system of determining the muscular structure of an individual head. As he put it:

The essence of the programme was that not only definite information about the thickness of the soft parts must be found, but also morphological features of the skull which could serve as clues for the reconstruction of the different parts of the face – nose, mouth, eyes and so forth.

Gerasimov spent two years measuring and dissecting the heads of corpses in the medical faculty of the university before attempting a reconstruction. He was disappointed with his first attempt, and showed it to no one. In 1925, however, he produced a portrait based on a contemporary skull which encouraged both him and Professor Grigoriev. That year he was appointed scientific technical assistant to the Irkutsk Museum, and was later put in charge of its archaeological section; there he reconstructed fossil heads, while at the same time persevering with his experiments on 'fleshed' heads.

It was not until 1935, 15 years after his first tentative steps had been taken, that an opportunity presented itself to prove to his colleagues that he was not driven by, as he put it, 'mania and fanaticism'. In the medical school he found the skeleton of a Dr Kolesnikov, who had left his body for research. Gerasimov had not known the doctor during his lifetime and had never seen a picture of him; however he was told that Kolesnikov's family had snapshots of him taken just before his death.

Carefully, Gerasimov set to work and produced on the skull the features of a man with a high, narrow forehead, a long nose, deep-set little eyes, a large though receding chin and protruding ears; despite this unprepossessing appearance Gerasimov judged that the muscular structure must have given the man a slightly smiling appearance, which 'lent the whole visage a surprising charm'. When Dr Kolesnikov's mother saw the reconstructed head she was at first shocked and then deeply moved; her collection of photographs showed the scientist how accurate he had been, and he presented the mother with the portrait.

The same year, Gerasimov's work received what at first he thought to be a setback. He was handed the skull of a Frenchman, one Loustalot, a famous boxer and fencing master who had taught athletics at Leningrad. Gerasimov constructed a likeness in his usual fashion, and then went to compare it with Loustalot's death mask, which was preserved at the Anatomical Institute in Leningrad. To his profound disappointment, only the forehead and twice-broken nose tallied with the death mask.

The whole of the lower part of the face was different and I would say even alien – strange. The face was noticeably broader, as though bloated. The blurred eyes projecting from their orbits and the swollen mouth with thick, shapeless lips were quite unlike those of the face modelled by me.

To Gerasimov's relief there was an explanation. Loustalot had dropped dead in the street, and some time passed before the body was identified. By the time his identity was established, decomposition was fairly advanced, though a death mask had been taken from the decaying features nonetheless. When the portrait was compared with pictures of Loustalot in life, it was found to be as accurate as Dr Kolesnikov's had been.

Professor Grigoriev was delighted with his pupil's progress, and in 1939 gave him his first criminological task. In a wood outside Leningrad numerous bones had been found, scattered over a fairly wide area. They bore the marks of animal teeth, and it was assumed that they were the remains of someone who had been attacked and killed by wolves. However the skull and lower jaw told a different tale; when Gerasimov examined it he found the marks of what he considered to be a small hunting hatchet, along with a fracture which had been made by a blunt instrument. Adhering to the crown were a number of reddish-blond hairs, which had been cut short some days before death.

The incomplete bone formation, the open sutures on the skull vault, the absence of wisdom teeth and the light wear on the adult teeth suggested to Gerasimov that the individual had been between twelve and thirteen years old. Sexing the head was difficult in view of the age, but the strongly developed supra-orbital region and the large mastoid processes among other features seemed to point to the victim having been a boy.

After carefully refitting the lower jaw into place, Gerasimov modelled the most important masticatory muscles – these determine the whole shape of the face. Little by little he remodelled the head taking into account such factors as the individual peculiarities in the relief of the skull, the nasal bones and the chin eminence. The result was a snub-nosed, chubby-cheeked boy with a high forehead, a thick upper lip and slightly projecting ears. Short, red-blond hair was finally added.

Meanwhile, the police had been searching their missing persons files for likely identities. Among them was a folio on a boy who, his parents believed, had run off to Leningrad six months previously. So as not to alarm them unduly, photographs of the reconstructed head were mixed in with 30 photographs of boys of similar age. The father immediately recognized the reconstruction as his son, and when the photograph was circulated the boy's movements were traced. As a result his attacker was caught and brought to trial: 'the first attempt to use a skull reconstruction in a criminal case was thus brilliantly successful' wrote Gerasimov, with justifiable pride.

Throughout the 1940s Gerasimov's fame grew in legal circles, and triumph followed triumph as his techniques became less empirical and more exact. Soon he was training students and by 1950 he had sufficient skilled pupils to establish his Laboratory for Plastic Reconstruction. With each case, he learned a little more about the morphology of the human face, but perhaps one final example suffices best to show how far he had come since his first tentative efforts in 1925.

Shortly after the setting up of the laboratory, Gerasimov was called upon to reconstruct the face of an elderly woman whose skeleton had been found in a hut in remote woodlands. About a year earlier, the wife of a forester had disappeared in odd circumstances; her husband had said that she had set off to visit their son in a neighbouring town, but had neither arrived at her destination nor returned home.

When Gerasimov examined the skull he found it severely damaged; the lower jaw was missing and only three molars in the upper jaw remained intact, the broken roots of the others remaining embedded in the skull. The roof of the mouth was peppered with small round holes, and in the base of the skull Gerasimov found several lead pellets. From this evidence he easily came to the conclusion that the woman had been killed by a shotgun blast from very close quarters.

Careful measuring of the remaining skull and comparison with other measurements in his files gave Gerasimov an idea of the shape of the missing lower jaw, and he was able to build this up in plaster, along with reconstructed teeth. His finished head resembled the missing wife so accurately that the forester confessed.

He had set out to drive his wife to their son's home in his horse-drawn wagon, but on the road there had been an argument. The forester had jumped from the wagon in a fury, telling his wife to drive herself; because the woods were haunted by wolves he had dragged down his double-barrelled shotgun from the back of the wagon, but in his irritation he mishandled the gun, and both barrels went off, one tearing away the bottom half of his wife's face, the other hitting her in the chest. In a panic he had hidden the body. After hearing his story and reconstructing the crime, police were convinced that he was telling the truth and he thus avoided a capital charge.

Despite Professor Gerasimov's success, Western criminologists have so far seldom followed the lead he has given – a fact which puzzles the more progressive among them. In the course of the past twenty years or so, the widespread use of such techniques as 'identikit' and 'photo-fit' to reconstruct the faces of wanted or missing persons from their description have made the processes familiar to the general public. They have also been used in the identification of corpses and there is little question that their effectiveness would be increased enormously were they to be taken in conjunction with the Gerasimov system.

What is perhaps even more extraordinary, in view of the testimony of such experts as Professor Keith Simpson, quoted earlier, is the fact that Western forensic odontology has lagged behind the work done by the Russians; Gerasimov attached great importance to teeth as a factor in criminal identification, and in fact the history of dental identification is ancient. Agrippina had an enemy killed, and satisfied herself that the right man had died by examining his teeth. In more recent years the victims of two disastrous fires – at the Vienna Opera House in 1878 and the Paris Charité in 1897 – were identified by their teeth. And yet one of Europe's few experts, Professor Gosta Gustafson, writing in the *Criminologist* magazine in 1969, had to

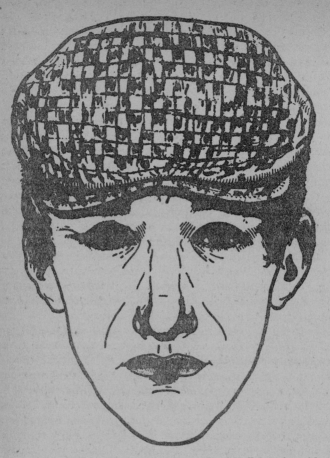

*A typical Identikit portrait, put together in collaboration with a witness, from a wide range of component features (Popperfoto).*

report that only three major forensic odontology departments existed in any of the world's dental schools – one in Norway, one in Denmark and one in Cuba.

Professor Simpson's interest in dental identification was aroused by one of his own cases, a classic of its kind. In July

1942, workmen demolishing an old Baptist chapel in the Lambeth district of London discovered the ossified, partly dismembered remains of a human being under the cellar floor. At first the body was thought to have been the result of a burial in the nearby churchyard, and even when preliminary examination showed that death had taken place between twelve and eighteen months previously, no immediate alarm was raised, the assumption being that it was the corpse of a bomb victim from the blitz.

However, when Professor Simpson had the body removed to his laboratory at Guy's Hospital and probed further, quite a different picture emerged. Lime had been strewn over the body; contrary to popular belief lime tends to preserve organic material, and in this case helped preserve the larynx, so that Professor Simpson was able to observe a fracture which suggested that death had been due to strangulation. Parts of the arms and legs, as well as the lower jaw, had been hacked away, and the flesh of the head had been removed in an attempt to avoid identification. A scrap of hair remained, however, and this and other evidence enabled a picture of the deceased to be built up. The body was that of a woman, aged between forty and fifty, five feet to five feet one inch tall, with dark brown hair going grey, in whose womb lay a fibroid tumour.

Police investigating the circumstances discovered that a man named Harry Dobkin had been a firewatcher at the Baptist chapel. Fifteen months previously his wife Rachel had disappeared after attempting to obtain maintenance arrears from him; on a previous occasion he had served a term of imprisonment for non-payment. Rachel Dobkin had been 47, five feet one inch in height, with dark brown hair going grey, and the records of two London hospitals showed that she had refused operations for a fibroid tumour of the womb. But proof of identity was essential to gain a conviction, and this data, strongly circumstantial though it was, was deemed to be insufficient.

Fortunately, the police were able to trace Mrs Dobkin's dentist, Barnet Kopkin of Crouch End, North London. Mr Kopkin produced the records of work he had done on Mrs Dobkin's upper jaw. His file and the jaw of the body were identical on five vital points: the number and position of the teeth, the situation of fillings, the marks of fitting a denture, the thickening of the weight bearing area of the molar sockets, and the remains of roots recorded as being left in the jaw. Harry Dobkin was convicted at the Old Bailey of murdering his wife and hanged.

Microscopic investigation of teeth in section reveals many things; the odontologist can establish whether or not the tooth is human and then proceed to give a fair estimation of the owner's age, state of health, and even occupation, habits and social position. A skilled and knowledgeable examiner can, says Professor Gustafson:

... trace the handiwork of a dentist in a certain country or even a certain dentist, because of characteristic details, individual to certain dental schools, but unknown or ignored by others.

Marks left by habits or occupation on the teeth are of two kinds, mechanical and chemical. Carpenters, upholsterers, cobblers and

## DESCRIPTION OF NUDE BODY OF MURDERED WOMAN

Found on Cutler Mountain, December 17th, 1904.

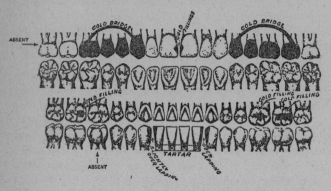

*Although attempts were made as early as 1904 to identify corpses by their teeth, the method is still not widely adopted.*

seamstresses tend to hold nails and needles between their teeth, and this practice eventually leaves marks. Wind musicians too, are quickly recognized by a forensic odontologist and even individual instruments can be identified – brass instruments such as the trumpet or trombone affect the teeth in one way, while woodwinds such as the clarinet or bassoon can also be distinguished. Workers in metals such as lead or copper develop chemical deposits on their teeth and gums, and smokers, of course, present many clues.

Cigarette smokers generally have smoke stains on the inner sides of the front teeth, while pipe smokers develop an irritation of the palate which shows up as a series of white rings with a red dot in the centre. The gripping of a pipe or cigarette holder between the teeth also leaves characteristic marks in wearing down the enamel.

There are small differences in the teeth of various races; Professor Gustafson points out, for instance, that the mongolian races – Chinese and Japanese – generally have characteristically shovel-shaped upper front teeth and a tendency to three-rooted lower back teeth, which seldom occur in other races.

Dental identification is particularly valuable in cases of death by fire, as the teeth tend to withstand intense heat better than any other part of the body, and dental experts are nowadays among the most important investigators in the case of plane crashes. Again, in the case of death by drowning, where the body has been immersed for a long period so that the skin of the hands has been sloughed off, teeth are invaluable.

But one of the most common uses of forensic odontology in actual crime comes in cases of sexual attack, where the attacker frequently bites his victim in a frenzy of lust. In a typical case investigated by Professor Gustafson, a young woman had been raped and murdered, and two men were suspected. On the dead woman's left breast were the clear impressions of a set of teeth, one of which had left a sharp scratch. The two men were examined. One of them had a gold filling in one of his upper incisors which had worn to a sharp edge; this fitted the wound on the breast exactly, as did the impression of his other teeth. He was tried and convicted on the evidence.

Again, in sexual cases, marks on the neck need to be clearly distinguished by the medical examiner. Where bruises are round, they have generally been made by fingertip pressure; an elliptical bruise usually indicates a 'love bite'.

That dental identification can also be aided by statistical investigation is shown by another remarkable case investigated by Professor Gustafson. The body of a young man was caught in the nets of a Swedish trawler in the Baltic Sea near the Danish island of Bornholm. The body was clad only in shorts, and had been in the water for some weeks. An examination of the teeth showed that they were in perfect condition apart from a single amalgam filling in one of the molars of the upper jaw.

As the body was found between the coasts of Germany, Sweden, Denmark and Russia, identification seemed at first to be a formidable task, but as a Danish vessel had been lost in the area some weeks before, records were collected from dentists who had treated known members of the crew, for comparison with the teeth of the unknown body. One dentist noted that he had made one filling in the mouth of a youth of about eighteen years, and had a record of the outline of the filling; he had also remarked on the file that this was the only work which had been done on the young man's teeth. Professor Gustafson wrote,

A previous investigation carried out on a great number of individuals in Malmö in Sweden had shown that this could be expected only once among about eight hundred boys and girls of the age of about fourteen years. At the age of 18 a maximum of only one filling is still more rare. The teeth from the body provided estimations of the age at the time of death. As it gave the result of about twenty years, it was considered without doubt that the body was that of the missing seaman from Denmark.

# Chapter Nine
# The mark of Cain

Death loves a shining mark, a signal blow.

Edward Young, *Night Thoughts*

The influence of Louis Quetelet's theory, that no two people can be identical, has continued over the years; today specialists in criminal science are considering such ideas as, for instance, that human lip prints may be as identifiable as fingerprints, and that recorded voice patterns can regularly convict criminals.

But even leaving aside these advanced ideas, Quetelet's theory has proved sound practice time and again over the past 150 years or so, as scientists discovered that, just as fingerprints and bone measurements were individual in character, so bodily distinguishing marks such as tattoos, scars, and blemishes could be pinpointed and if necessary used against their owners.

From the criminologists' point of view, for instance, the presence of tattooing on a suspect or a body is extremely helpful. The scars are virtually inerradicable, and yet the so-called 'criminal classes' appear always to have favoured tattooing as personal decoration, thus making the task of their hunters so much easier. Roman slaves were tattooed by their owners, and the marks remained even if they escaped or were freed.

But it was among the sailors, and to a lesser extent soldiers, of eighteenth-century England that tattooing came into its own; and many of these men were forced by the hardships of service life to desert and thus become wanted criminals. Some ships' captains recorded details of tattoo marks among their crews in the ship's log, in order to make identification easier if a man jumped ship. A favourite design among wrong-doers in the British Navy of the time was a crucifix emblazoned across the shoulder blades: superstition held that the thongs of the cat o' nine tails would cringe from striking the sacred image.

Criminals in Napoleonic France were either less superstitious or more confident than their counterparts across the Channel and, as the use of the guillotine spread after the Revolution, took to having dotted lines tattooed around their necks, with the inscription 'cut here'. This particular piece of bravado has remained popular with French criminals ever since.

Most professional tattooists today use insoluble pigments, working the design into the lower layers of skin with a needle. To obscure the design later is a difficult task, even if soluble inks have been used; another pattern may be tattooed on top of the original, but ultraviolet and infra-red photography show up such deceits immediately. Even treatment with chemical caustics or by electrolysis – two of the most common methods of erasing tattoo work – leave scars in the surrounding lymph glands which when magnified or, in the case of a post-mortem, dissected, are instantly apparent.

So to all intents and purposes the tattoo, once made, is permanent, and perhaps for this reason as much as any other has become a favourite feature of fictional crime story writers. What is a fact is that tattoos have turned up as evidence in real life crime in the most bizarre ways: perhaps the best known case was that of the Sydney shark.

On 25 April 1935, a shark in the Coogee Aquarium, Sydney, which had been netted a week earlier, went berserk. The fourteen-foot creature began dashing from side to side of the pool, thrashing around in the water, and finally vomited up the contents of its stomach: these included a human arm. The shark died and a post-mortem examination of it revealed no more pieces of human tissue; the arm had obviously been swallowed before the creature's capture the week before, and normally its strong intestinal juices would have digested the flesh in just over a day. However, fishery experts found indications that it had been upset by its change of environment and that as a result it had suffered from indigestion, and its gastric processes had slowed almost to a standstill.

Even odder coincidences were to come; the arm was tattooed with a rather rare design in the form of two boxes squaring up to each other. Sydney police quickly discovered that the description fitted only one man on their missing files, a billiard hall worker named James Smith, who had left home to go on a fishing expedition on 8 April, nine days before the shark's capture.

According to Smith's wife, who identified the disgorged limb, the tattoo was the only distinguishing peculiarity of his body. Furthermore, Smith's prints were on file, and the police were able to confirm the identification through them.

Forensic experts were now faced with the question of whether or not Smith was alive or dead. His death could not automatically be assumed, for many living people had lost limbs in the shark-infested waters of Sydney Harbour and Bondi beach. However, a length of rope had been tied around the wrist of the arm, and pathologists established that the severing, near the shoulder, was the work of a sharp instrument rather than a shark bite. Furthermore there were indications that the arm had been severed some time after death.

Two men were arrested and charged with the murder of Smith, but due to several technicalities they were acquitted the following September. For one thing the Australian Supreme Court ruled that an inquest could only be held on a body: an arm was not enough. This decision, incidentally, has since been revoked. The prosecution surmised, however, from several pieces of evidence before them, that Smith had been killed, dismembered, and packed in a weighted trunk. Only the arm would not fit in the trunk, and had been tied on outside before the whole package was taken out to sea and sunk. Ironically, the arm was the only part of the body which bore a distinguishing mark, and it had been swallowed by the one shark out of hundreds in the area destined to be captured for an aquarium within hours. And the final coincidence was that this shark had suffered from a complaint almost unknown among its kind – indigestion.

What was described by a senior police officer as 'an incredible' tattoo coincidence led to the arrest of Richard Franklin Speck, who was convicted in April 1967 of the cold-blooded slaughter of eight student nurses in a hostel in Chicago's Southside area. On 14 July 1966, Speck entered the hostel on East 100th Street, apparently with intent to rob, but instead stabbed eight of the residents to death. It was a particularly motiveless act, for no attempt to molest the nurses sexually was made, and only a few dollars were on the premises. Through an oversight on the part of the killer one girl, Corazon Amurao, managed to hide and give the police a rough description of the attacker. Local papers described it as 'Chicago's Crime of the Century' and the police, led by Detective Sergeant John Murtaugh, were quick to act. Through a clever series of deductions, Murtaugh surmised that the wanted man had at some time been a sailor, and within a few hours had a United States Coastguard file before him – a file which bore Speck's name. Also on the file was the information that Speck's body was tattooed in several places, including a serpent and the words 'Born to Raise Hell' on one forearm.

For various reasons, Murtaugh had not yet released a photograph or full description of the killer to the press; the principal reason was that he had a lead on Speck, and did not want to alarm him before it was followed through.

Police interviewed residents in the district, showing them Speck's portrait. On their seventh or eighth call they came upon Mrs Jo Holland, who lived on the twelfth floor of a high rise apartment block. Mrs Holland was a widow, and frequently occupied her time watching the street below through a pair of high-powered binoculars. She told police that early on the morning following the murder she had been seated at her post when a cab had stopped below, out of which had come a young man who resembled the one in the photograph shown her by the police.

'Then,' as Murtaugh said later, 'she delivered her blockbuster. She said that the early sunlight was so clear that she spotted a snake tatoo on the guy's forearm, and had been able to read the inscription on it: "Born to Raise Hell".'

The police dragnet closed on the area, and Speck was arrested, after trying to commit suicide, just 67 hours from the time of the first alarm. At his trial he pleaded not guilty, and it was not until February 1978, his death sentence commuted to life imprisonment, that he confessed and gave a full account of the murders.

Like tattoos, scars, made either accidentally or through a medical operation, are permanent, though sometimes they may be invisible to the naked eye, and due to the fact that they are composed of fibrous tissue may alter shape over a period as the tissue contracts. To some extent their age can be calculated by experts, though not always with absolute accuracy. Nevertheless, scars have provided evidence in many a criminal case, and a scar was a major factor in sending the notorious Dr Crippen to the gallows.

The outline of the Crippen case is fairly well known; Hawley Harvey Crippen, a graduate of the American teaching hospital system, had arrived in Britain in 1900, with his wife, Cora Crippen, a small-time music-hall singer. Because he was disqualified from practising as a physician in Britain with only an American diploma, Crippen operated on the dubious fringes of medicine for several years, peddling patent cures, while his wife, under the stage name Cora Belle Elmore, tried fairly unsuccessfully to establish herself as a singer on the London vaudeville circuit.

On the evening of 31 January 1910, Cora was seen with her husband at their home in Hilldrop Crescent, North London, but was never seen alive thereafter. Police, suspicious of Crippen's story that she had gone to relatives in California, made enquiries and found that Crippen had been having an affair with his secretary, a girl named Ethel Le Neve. For several months the little doctor bluffed and blustered, and finally fled the country under the name of Robinson, taking Ethel with him disguised as his 'son' aboard the passenger liner SS *Montrose*. The ship was bound for Canada, but the captain recognized the 'Robinsons' and sent a radio message back to London, and Scotland Yard's Chief Inspector Walter Dew was able to catch a faster vessel than the *Montrose* and be in the St Lawrence river to arrest the couple when they docked. It was, of course, the first time that the 'wireless' had been used to catch a murderer.

But, for forensic experts, the real drama was yet to come. Digging in the basement of Crippen's house, police had found a mass of human flesh; the limbs and head were missing, as were both the internal and external sexual organs. The heart, a lung, the oesophagus and stomach, liver, kidneys, and pancreas were the only other organs identifiable. Most grisly of all, the carcass had been 'boned' by what appeared to be a skilled medical hand.

Dr Augustus Joseph Pepper, who held the official title of Home Office pathologist and was perhaps the leading exponent of forensic medicine in the world, was given charge of the hideous remains. One of the first things he noticed was what appeared to

165

be a section of scar tissue between four and five inches long, slightly thickened at one end, which lay in what seemed to be a piece of flesh from the abdomen. Pepper handed over the segment of flesh to Dr Bernard Spilsbury, who was then 33 years old and Senior Pathologist at St Mary's Hospital.

From a few strands of longish hair found at the site, along with what appeared to be a woman's vest, the possibility that the remains were those of a female seemed strong, but this was not for Spilsbury to surmise. He worked long and hard at his evidence before the trial opened on 18 October 1910.

It became obvious that the principal defence that could be put forward on Crippen's behalf would be that the sections of the torso were not those of a woman at all, and that they had been buried without Crippen's knowledge, probably before he took the house the previous autumn.

Accordingly, the defence solicitor asked Hubert Turnbull, a pathologist at the London Hospital and a rival of Pepper and Spilsbury, to examine the tissue bearing the scar. In court, Turnbull claimed firstly that the piece of flesh he had seen had not come from the abdominal area because of the absence from it of certain tendons. Secondly, the 'scar' was merely a fold in the flesh, formed by the pressure upon it. It could not, he maintained, be a scar because no needle punctures from the sutures could be detected, and because parts of the sebaceous glands and fat corpuscles, which would not be present in the fibrous tissue of a true scar, were present.

Spilsbury answered calmly but dramatically. With a forceps, he pointed out the 'missing' tendon to the judge and jury; shamefacedly, Turnbull had to admit that he had not noticed it. Then, using microscopic slides, Spilsbury showed how the sebaceous glands and fat corpuscles, along with a few hair follicles, had been folded slightly into the scar during the suturing of the wound. In his opinion, said Spilsbury, the scar had been formed as the result of a hysterectomy operation; and Cora Crippen had undergone such an operation some time before coming to England.

This evidence was final damnation for the Crippen case, the prosecution having already shown that the woman's body had contained a lethal dose of the vegetable drug hyoscine, and that

Crippen had recently bought a quantity of the drug. Crippen went to the gallows and the first major triumph for forensic histology (the study of organic tissues) had been brought about.

It was not that scar evidence had not been used before in courts of law, but that few people seemed to understand the nature of scar tissue. A scar became a key factor as early as 1805, in New York, when an innocent man named Joseph Parker escaped a jail sentence for not supporting a woman named Catherine Hoag and her daughter – after she had claimed that he was her missing husband, Thomas Hoag.

Thomas Hoag, a carpenter, had married the woman Catherine in 1800 and had lived happily with her and their baby daughter until the child was three, when he suddenly vanished. One day in 1805, Mrs Hoag spotted a man whom she swore was her husband, challenged him, and was 'confirmed' in her suspicions when she heard his voice, which had a lisp. She had him arrested, though he swore that he was Joseph Parker.

Brought to court, each side summoned witness after witness; for Parker, several said that he had lived near them on the outskirts of the city since the 1790s, and had never left home. Against him, several more pointed out that Hoag had had a horseshoe-shaped scar on his forehead, and a wen on his neck, and sure enough Parker had both of these. In all 14 witnesses took the stand, seven with seemingly irrefutable evidence against Parker, and seven with equally sound evidence in his favour. Then Mrs Hoag's last witness appeared. He said that the man in the dock was definitely Hoag, because he had known him since childhood; indeed he had once saved his life by staunching the blood from a huge wound on the sole of Hoag's foot after he had accidentally stepped on a sharp knife. Somewhat wearily, the judge asked the defendant to take off his boots; both feet were unblemished, and he was allowed to go free.

One of the most disturbing cases of mistaken identity occurred in England at the end of the nineteenth century, during which something rather more than mere scar tissue was ignored by the prosecution. It began in 1877, when a man named Joseph Smith was arrested on charges of having seduced and defrauded 17 women of money and jewellery. A number of the women recognized him as the man who, calling himself 'Lord Salisbury',

'Lord Wilton' or 'Lord Willoughby', had wormed his way into their hearts and their bank accounts. He received four years imprisonment, was released in 1881, and vanished.

In December 1896 a respectable Norwegian mine owner named Adolf Beck was stopped in London by a woman who accused him of having stolen watches and rings from her after introducing himself as 'Lord Salisbury'. The police were called and, vehemently denying everything, Beck was arrested, charged, and placed in a police line-up while the officers in the case brought in 22 women who had laid similar charges, during the past few years, of being defrauded in the same manner. All but one positively identified Beck, a grey-haired, elderly man with a handlebar moustache, as their false lover. Despite his protests that he had been in South America in 1877, when Joseph Smith had been arrested, the prosecution alleged that Smith and Beck were one and the same, and Beck served five years of a seven years' hard labour sentence.

In 1910 he came out of jail, determined to prove his innocence. He had, while in jail, petitioned to be allowed to see Smith's record, and he had been refused. At that time there was no Court of Criminal Appeal, so Beck, now impoverished, had to seek what evidence he could alone. Then, on 15 April 1904, fate dealt what at the time must have seemed a further cruel blow. He was accosted in the street by a young woman and accused, exactly as before, of having swindled her. As if in a nightmare, Beck accompanied the woman and a policeman to Paddington police station where he was again accused by five women of being the bogus 'Lord'. On 27 June, Beck again appeared at the Old Bailey where he was convicted the same day. The judge deferred sentence, and Beck was held in custody at Paddington before being sent to prison. On 7 July, ten days later, Detective Inspector Kane, who had been involved in aspects of the Beck case, called at Tottenham Court Road police station on a routine matter. An officer there mentioned that a swindler had been brought in that afternoon, after trying to sell rings he had stolen from two actresses. When Kane saw the prisoner he was appalled to find himself looking at the double of Adolf Beck. The man called himself William Thomas.

Kane immediately sent to Scotland Yard for Joseph Smith's

record, for the details of Beck's pleas in court were still fresh in his mind. The file contained two items damning, not only to Smith-alias-Thomas but to the British judicial system of the time. Smith had a large scar under his ear and was circumcised. Beck had no scar, and was uncircumcised: a curious detail in view of the fact that he was alleged to have seduced over thirty of the embezzled women. Thomas fitted Smith's record exactly in physical detail, and when the female witnesses were confronted with him they admitted that they had been mistaken in naming Beck: Smith-Thomas was in reality the man who had robbed them. Even more shamefacedly they admitted that their joint seducer had lacked a foreskin: they had not thought to mention this 'indelicate' fact before.

Smith went to jail for a long term. Adolf Beck was granted a free pardon on both charges for which he had been convicted, and was awarded the somewhat derisory sum of £5000 compensation. The most important outcome of the affair was the setting up of the British Court of Criminal Appeal, so that poor Beck's false imprisonment served some purpose after all.

The case seems to have impressed the detective fiction writer Dorothy L. Sayers, and some years afterwards she is reported to have tried to introduce circumcision as an identifying feature into one of her stories; but despite her status and popularity at the time, she was forbidden by her publishers to do so.

While scars, tattoos and other such body marks as moles and birthmarks lack the positive weight of fingerprints as evidence, they can, taken in conjunction with other factors, supply vital circumstantial leads during the course of an investigation – in fact in the early stages they can be more important than fingerprints in establishing an overall picture.

Forensic experts look, Sherlock Holmes-fashion, for 'occupational' marks on the body; coal miners, for instance, are usually 'tattooed' minutely by fragments of coal which have been driven under the skin of the face over the years and show as small blue spots. The callouses of their hands too, are often ingrained with coal dust. Similarly, painters, metal workers, and engineers bear almost ineradicable traces of their occupations under the skin of their hands.

Stringed instrument players have extremely individual marks;

besides callouses on the tips of the left fingers and the inside of the thumb, the fingernails of a banjo picker or classical guitarist's right hand will be longer than those of his left. Bricklayers suffer flattening and hardening of the thumb and index finger on the hand they use for picking up bricks, while cobblers, seamstresses, and sail-makers tend to have roughened left index fingers, accompanied by minute diagonal scars caused by the twine, waxed thread, or cotton. Writers and secretaries tend to have slightly hardened tips on at least the first three fingers of each hand – a good touch typist will have them on all eight fingers – while those who habitually use a pen grow a thickening on the first knuckle of the middle finger. While useful, these bodily indications are indications only, and most experts prefer to back them up with other corroboration.

Dr Joseph Bell was a surgeon at the Edinburgh Royal Infirmary and lectured the young Arthur Conan Doyle while Doyle was a medical student there. Bell was Doyle's model for Sherlock Holmes; his methods of deduction, not only during an autopsy but while interviewing live patients, were sometimes uncanny, until they were explained – exactly as Holmes's in fiction. It is said that it was Bell who used the phrase 'Elementary, my dear Doyle' when his young student was baffled; Holmes, in fact, never uses exactly that phrase in his books.

The distinguished forensic pathologist Sir Sydney Smith learned much from the legends of Dr Bell, heard at Edinburgh when he too was a student there, though Bell had died some years before. On one occasion, Smith was told by an eyewitness, Dr Bell glanced casually at a patient as he came through the door and said: 'Good morning. You are a left-handed cobbler.'

The man, and Bell's students, were astounded at his accuracy. Bell explained that the worn places on the thighs of the man's trousers could only have been made by a lapstone, and that the right side was more worn than the left because he hammered the leather with his left hand.

But even the prodigious Bell was aware of the dangers of unsupported deduction, as he liked to illustrate in a story he told against himself. Bell was taking a group of students in the outpatients department of the Infirmary when a man came through the door. Bell walked around him, and then announced that he was a recently discharged soldier who had served for a long period in the East in the Royal Scots regiment and had played the euphonium in the regimental band.

He explained to the students that the soldier had stood rigidly to attention when he first came in, and then relaxed. 'No civilian ever does that, and a soldier, after he has been discharged for some time, also neglects to do so. Hence I deduced that he had probably not long been discharged from the Army.'

Bell also pointed out the deep tanning of the man's face and neck, and the oriental-style tattoo on his arm, and the fact that he was wearing a belt with the Royal Scots buckle, which suggested that he had been in that regiment. But he was a little short for the regular infantry of the time, so that he was probably in the band. If so he had played the euphonium:

If you look at his chest and observe the way he breathes you will note that he shows all the signs of emphysema [dilation of the air vessels in the lungs] which may well be due to playing a large wind instrument: hence my suggestion that he had been a player of such an instrument for many years.

Turning to the patient, Bell confidently asked had he been a soldier? Yes, replied the man. In the Royal Scots? Yes. For long? Twenty years, in India. In the band? All the time.

'And of course you played the euphonium?' asked Bell with a flourish towards his students.

'No sir,' replied the old soldier impassively. 'The big drum sir.'

It is almost certainly true that Louis Quetelet was correct in all essentials when he said that no two human beings could be totally alike, even leaving aside fingerprints. Suggestions have been made – very tentatively – that the veins on the backs of the hands, the stomach, and even the breath are as individual as the loops, whorls and ridges on the human hands and feet. True or false, the great advantage which fingerprints possess over all these is ease of classification. Until the unlikely day when criminologists can note and classify and place on file such details, the circumstantial evidence offered by scars, tattoos, moles and other body marks will remain invaluable to the forensic expert.

# Chapter Ten
# Hanging by a hair

*Other things are all very well in their way,
but give me Blood!*

Charles Dickens, *David Copperfield*

During his forty-plus years of work in police coroners' courts, the opinion of Sir Bernard Spilsbury was rarely totally disregarded. On numerous occasions the opposition attempted to counter his testimony, but perhaps only in the case of George Margerison was it ignored altogether by two juries, for reasons that will perhaps never be known.

George Margerison was 16 years old, the son of a middle-class family who lived at Ribchester, Lancashire, and who was, in Spilsbury's own words, a 'normal, healthy boy'. In March 1926 he was found dead in a secluded lane near his home, shot through the head with a .32 Mauser automatic. An inquest was held, and the jury returned the verdict of suicide.

The Margerison family was dissatisfied, however, and George's father applied to the King's Bench Division of the High Court for a second inquest, the motion being granted. Mr Margerison also wrote to Sir Bernard asking if he would view his son's body, and Spilsbury agreed. He examined the corpse with a local police surgeon, and came to the conclusion which he announced at the second inquest in September: 'By whatever means the boy came by his death it was not suicide.'

To Spilsbury's astonishment, the jury again returned a verdict of suicide. Spilsbury was so annoyed that he gathered evidence, including the boy's bowler hat, made several experiments, and then prepared a lecture on the case which he gave to several prominent gatherings of medico-legal men.

The basic facts were straightforward. George Margerison was found lying on the ground with an entrance wound in his right temple and an exit wound above and behind the left ear; on the face of it the classic path taken by a suicide's bullet. However, there were no marks whatsoever around the entrance wound; no singeing of the hair, no powder 'tattoo' marks, no blackening of the flesh or 'rebound' bruises, which clearly indicated that the shot had been fired from some distance. Futhermore, the weapon lay on the left of the body, near the left hand, while the bullet had entered from the right, and clenched between the fingers of the boy's left hand was the stub of a partly smoked cigarette.

But the hat itself, which had lain brim down on the body's left, had its own tale to tell. The bowler was spattered with tiny spots of blood over the outer right-hand surface and extending forward and downward under the curve of the brim. Large bloodstains had splashed onto the inside leather lining in a right to left direction; while spattered blood and brain matter were found under the brim on the left-hand side.

As Spilsbury himself observed in his notes, the presence of blood on the hat showed that it was on the boy's head when he was shot, and the two wounds of entrance and exit must have been close under the brim. A bullet passing through the skull produces a tremendous pressure during the estimated $\frac{1}{500}$ of a second that it takes to traverse the cranial cavity, and this pressure forces out blood through the entrance wound; when the fine spray of blood meets the gases discharged from the gun it is blown back to the surface of the head. In this case it had stained the hat. The bloodstains on the inner lining, said Spilsbury, indicated 'that the gases also raised the hat from the head', and the bullet as it emerged from the left side of the head spattered blood and brain spray on the bowler's brim on that side too.

The fact that the boy kept the hat on ran counter to most examples of head-shot suicide that Spilsbury knew. For psychological reasons the suicide planning his own death in this way removes his head gear; and that fact coupled with the position of the gun and the cigarette butt in the left hand brought Spilsbury to the conclusion that suicide must be ruled out. But if the case was murder, it was never solved.

In his notes on the Margerison case, Sir Bernard Spilsbury remarked:

The bloodstain on the undersurface of the brim of the left side no doubt followed the bullet as it emerged from the head. This result from the passage of a bullet through the head has not been recorded previously as far as I can ascertain.

In fact at that time the study of serology had advanced very little since 1628, when the physician Sir William Harvey discovered the circulation of the blood. The word serology comes from the Sanskrit word *sara* – 'to flow' – and today the forensic medical examiner knows that not only blood but semen, saliva, and any other body substance which 'flows' can be of value in a criminal investigation, not only to convict the guilty but to clear the innocent.

Observers such as Eugene Vidocq and Alexandre Lacassagne noted the shapes adopted by blood spots when they fell. Glaister gives six categories of these – drops, smears, splashes, spurts, trails, and pools. Circular drops, for instance, indicate that the blood has fallen directly onto the surface on which it is found. Blood landing from an angle causes an 'exclamation mark' stain, the shape of which indicates the direction from which it has come and the velocity at which it was travelling. A blow on the head can either produce a circular drop or an exclamation mark stain, depending on the position of the body at the time of the assault.

Smears, trails, and pools are self evident in their origin; if a freshly wounded body is moved it will leave a dribble of blood along the course taken, and usually a pool of blood at the point at which it is deposited. Bloody finger smears on a wall, for instance – though unlikely to yield usable fingerprints – can be analysed to show whether the blood is that of the victim or of attacker. Although detailed photographs of the scene of a violent crime are taken by police photographers, if a pictorial record of bloodstain distribution is required an artist will be called in to prepare a plan showing in particular the size, shape and position of the bloodstains.

Glaister points out the dangers of premature assumption in cases where what appear to be bloodstains are present. Blood changes colour under differing circumstances; the age of the stain, the amount of blood present, the nature and colour of the material on which it falls, and attempts to wash it off or otherwise eliminate it, all alter the appearance of bloodstains. The age of a bloodstain cannot be accurately assessed at the time of writing, but broadly speaking fresh blood is bright red and turns first to a rust colour, and then to chocolate brown as it ages.

Many substances produce blood-like stains, including various jams, fruit juices (particularly banana juice), chocolate, vegetable dyes, rust and snuff, but a quick preliminary test enables these to be distinguished from a true bloodstain. From examination of the apparel of the victim, the examiner can get a first-hand idea of how and from what direction the blood was spilled. Had this procedure been carried out in the case of Dr Sam Sheppard of Ohio, both distress to Sheppard and expense to the state might have been avoided.

In 1954, Sam Sheppard was 30, and had already made a name for himself as a brilliant neurosurgeon. He was the youngest son of Dr Richard A. Sheppard, a general surgeon and osteopath who had founded the Bay View Hospital at Cleveland, Ohio, where Sam and his father and two elder brothers, Richard and Stephen, worked. Nine years previously, he had married pretty Marilyn Reese, and the couple lived in a fashionable and expensive four-bedroomed house on the shores of Lake Erie, which had a private beach. They were an apparently happy and popular pair.

On the night of 3 July 1954, a Mr and Mrs Ahern were guests for dinner at the Sheppard house, and they reported later that the meal was pleasantly convivial, though the doctor seemed a little tired. After dinner the Sheppard's young son Chip was put to bed, and the adults poured drinks and settled down to watch television. By midnight, however, Sam Sheppard had fallen asleep in his chair, and by half past twelve, Mrs Sheppard was showing her guests out.

Subsequent events were undeniably vague, and there was only one witness to them: Dr Sam himself. According to his story, which never varied in the slightest during the coming years, he was awakened by the sound of Marilyn's screams, coming from upstairs. He dashed up to the bedroom, and was hit from behind. When he came to, he realized that she was 'in a very bad condition'. Dazedly, he ran to his son's bedroom, but Chip was still sleeping and unharmed. Then he heard a noise downstairs, and ran down in time to see a shadowy figure run from the back door and make for the beach. He gave chase, managed to grab at the figure, but was again knocked unconscious. This time when he awoke he was lying half in and half out of the lake, dripping wet, and dressed only in trousers and shoes; the T shirt he had been wearing after dinner had gone.

It was now 5.45 am. Sheppard staggered back to the house in a horror-stricken daze, ascertained that his wife was dead, and rang his friend and near neighbour, local mayor J. Spencer Houk.

'For God's sake Spen, come quick! I think they've got Marilyn.' Houk arrived quickly, followed by the police, Dr Richard Sheppard, and the coroner, Dr Samuel Gerber. The scene they found in the bedroom was one of exceptional violence. Mrs Sheppard had been hit on the head 35 times with a 'blunt instrument' and her blood covered the bedclothes and pillow thickly, as well as having been spattered about the walls and furniture. Her body was clad only in a pyjama top, which had been pulled up over her breasts, and her legs dangled over the edge of the bed. Dr Gerber estimated the time of death at between 3 and 4 am.

There was some evidence that Gerber was jealous of the success of the Sheppard family in local medicine. At the final Sheppard trial, evidence was brought in that some months before the killing he had boasted that 'he would get the Sheppards' one day. His reply was 'Anyone who says that is a liar!'

Nevertheless it was through his testimony at the first trial, which lasted from October to December 1954, and was then the longest murder trial in American history, that Sheppard was convicted of second degree murder and sentenced to life. Samuel Gerber led the investigation from the start, and his very first act on arriving at the murder house was to point out to the police that the ransacked drawers and cupboards could have been a clumsy attempt to make the killing look like the act of a burglar. Where was Dr Sam's missing T shirt? Why had his medical bag been turned upside down on the floor with a box of morphine ampoules missing? Searching the grounds of the house, police found a canvas bag, which Sheppard used on his boat, lying under some bushes. It contained Sam's bloodstained watch, his fraternity ring, and the key ring and chain which normally hung from his belt. It could have been left there by the attacker, admitted Gerber, but could it not also have been put there by Sheppard in an attempt to put the police off the scent?

This question was never answered, and several more were never asked, either by prosecution or defence. For instance fibres were found under Marilyn's finger-nails. They were not apparently from Sheppard's clothing, but no one questioned their presence further. Nor was the fact that a tooth chipped from the dead woman's mouth was almost certainly the result of her having bitten hard into her attacker, and broken it off as he dragged away. The result would have left a nasty tear, but there were no bite or scratch marks on Sheppard's body.

As these investigations went on, Gerber reported them to the local press, which published them in full. He also announced the discovery that the doctor had been having an extramarital affair with a young woman colleague. These factors, and Gerber's claim that an imprint on Mrs Sheppard's pillow could 'only have been made by a surgical instrument' sealed the doctor's fate.

For the next twelve years Sheppard languished in jail, but he was rarely out of the news as his attorney fought to get him a re-trial on the grounds of press pre-trial prejudice. Eventually he secured the services of an astute young Boston lawyer, F. Lee Bailey. It was through Bailey's efforts that the United States Supreme Court quashed the conviction for murder and ordered a re-trial, which began on October 24 1966, with Lee Bailey leading the defence.

Bailey's cross examination of the investigating officer in the case, Sergeant Robert Schottke, embarrassed the policeman and impressed the court from the start. Had Schottke realized that the killer must have left prints on the watch, key chain, and ring found in Dr Sheppard's canvas duffle bag, and if so had he tested them for prints? In a low voice Schottke admitted that he had not. And what about the injuries which Sheppard had suffered to the back of his head – had it been proved or disproved by independent medical evidence whether or not they could have been self-inflicted? The sergeant admitted again that such evidence had not been sought.

Bailey next attacked Gerber, bringing in the evidence that he had wanted to 'get' the Sheppard family. Gerber's blustering reply caused a silence to fall on the courtroom. In the hush, Bailey asked him about the bloody imprint of a 'surgical instrument' on the pillow. Could Gerber describe what he had in mind? No, was the answer. Had he ever found such an instrument? Again the answer was no.

But at this point, Gerber counter-attacked. He showed colour transparencies of the watch and other items found in the duffle sailing bag. The watch face was spattered with flecks of blood which could, he argued, only have got there while the accused was beating his wife to death. For a time, Bailey was baffled. The entire case seemed to hang on the 'flying blood' evidence. And then a fresh thought struck him. He ordered blown up copies of the transparencies to be made; they showed the splattered watch face, but they also showed the inside of the watch band too, and that also bore blood 'freckles'. The blood must, therefore have got onto the watch after it had been removed from Sam Sheppard's wrist and, as he had been wearing it at dinner that night, it must have been removed after he was beaten over the head for the first time: when, in fact, he ran to help his screaming wife and interrupted her killer.

'The prosecution's case,' Bailey summed up, 'is ten pounds of hogwash in a five pound bag.' The jury agreed, and Sheppard was declared not guilty. Sadly for Sheppard, public opinion, turned against him twelve years before, was reflected in the attitude of the medical authorities. It took him more than a year to have his name restored to the medical roll, and even then business was not brisk. He took to professional wrestling for a living and eventually died, disillusioned by his rejection, in April 1970.

Of course, not only the shape and direction of bloodstains are considered by crime investigators; blood is classifiable into groups, and to a certain extent group classification as far as forensic serology is concerned is a negative factor. Large numbers of grouping systems are available today which can be used to positively eliminate but only rarely to identify someone, as any one combination of blood groups will almost certainly occur in many individuals in a given population.

178

As Alistair R. Brownlie, Solicitor to the Supreme Courts of Edinburgh, put it to the British Forensic Society:

Since Cain slew Abel, spilt blood has borne its mute testimony in crimes of violence. Stains of blood and body fluids still play an important part in crime detection, a lesser but increasing part in the proof of guilt.

A classic example of the latter concept occurred just under eleven years after the Sheppard case in the village of East Harland, Litchfield County, Connecticut, a small community peopled by Norwegian settlers. On 15 June 1965, bookkeeper Arnfin Thompsen returned home to find his wife Dottie lying dead in a great pool of her own blood. Police Chief O'Brien sent for the chief toxicologist for the state of Connecticut, Dr Abraham Stolman, and together they began the investigation. Stolman noted the violence with which the murder had been carried out. The dead woman's face had been entirely crushed in, her jaw smashed, and her left temple pulped. A thick smear of blood led from the enclosed porch, on which she was found, back into the house and through into the kitchen. In a corner of the kitchen stood Dottie's ironing board, and it was here that she appeared to have been killed; a white skirt which she had apparently been ironing was spattered, and blood covered the floor, walls and furniture.

Obviously the blows which had killed Mrs Thompsen had been delivered with great force, and equally obviously the killer must have been smeared with gore when the deed was done. The only other occupant of the Thompsen house was the dead woman's mother-in-law, Agnes Thompsen. She lived in a self-contained apartment on the top floor of the stone and clapboard cottage, and when visited by the police acted with strange equanimity.

'Is she dead yet?' she asked calmly, when she caught sight of her daughter-in-law's shrouded body. Agnes Thompsen's son Arnfin told the investigating officers that his mother, a widow, was a religious fanatic whose fanaticism had, in fact, overstepped the bounds. She had recently spent almost a year in the Connecticut Valley Hospital for the mentally ill, and, though released, her mind was failing steadily. But could this frail old woman have wrought such violence? Chief O'Brien, perhaps with memories of the adage which holds that the insane 'have 'the strength of ten', thought she could. Although a perfunctory search of her apartment showed no signs of bloodstains, either on her clothing or elsewhere, she had had, he pointed out to Dr Stolman, plenty of time to clean up if she had committed the murder; the body had apparently been killed earlier in the day.

Stolman, like the professional medical examiner he was, preferred to keep an open mind. Traces of blood were found in the kitchen sink trap – the pipe which leads from the plug hole – which suggested that someone had washed there. There was also a bloodstained dress in a linen closet – out of the line of any splashing – which could have been used by the killer to wipe away evidence. After experimenting, however, Dr Stolman decided that the blood in the sink had probably got there during the murder; and the blood on the dress was an old stain. All the blood in the house was Mrs Thompsen's, according to group testing.

Then came an apparently damning discovery. On checking through Agnes Thompsen's apartment more methodically, a brown stain which looked like blood was found on the stairway leading up to it; vigorous attempts had been made to scrub the wood clean. Dr Stolman had the whole stair removed and subjected to analysis, only to find that it was Agnes Thompsen's own blood, which was of a different group from that of her daughter-in-law. No other traces of any kind were found in Agnes's rooms, and it became obvious that the feeble-minded old woman had only reacted as she did because of her mental state. In the end a routine check of the village uncovered the the real culprit – a neighbour of the Thompsens who had borne a grudge.

The basic principles of the 'typing' of blood were first discovered in 1900 by the Viennese doctor Karl Landsteiner, who received a Nobel Prize for his work in serology in 1930. Subsequent developments have made the subject increasingly complex, but it is still possible to describe the principles in a simplified way.

When blood is exposed to the air it separates into a solid clot and liquid serum, the clot containing all the blood cells, white and red. The red cells each carry a number of antigens, substances which stimulate the production of antibodies to fight disease, and which will also react with certain specific antibodies. These antibodies are in the blood serum.

Landsteiner discovered that the blood of all humans could be divided into one of four types depending on the presence or absence of two antigens in the red cells. The antigens are called A and B and the corresponding antibodies in the serum are called anti-A and anti-B. The four types are:

Group A – antigen A and antibody B present (B and anti-A absent)

Group B – antigen B and antibody A present (A and anti-B absent)

Group O – antigens A and B absent, antibodies A and B present

Group AB – antigens A and B present, antibodies A and B absent

If two different types of blood were mixed, a clumping together of the red cells occurred which was visible to the naked eye. Cells of type A showed clumping when mixed with serum of type B or O; cells of type B showed clumping when mixed with serum of type A or O and cells of type AB showed clumping when mixed with serum of all three types. Only cells from type O blood could be mixed with serum from the other three. From this simple procedure a method for typing blood was soon developed. Drops of the blood to be typed were placed in slight depressions in an opal-glass plate, and drops of different types of serum were added to each. According to the clumping that took place, the blood could be immediately identified as A, B, O or AB. The type of blood found in a child follows the normal laws of inheritance, the genes for types A and B being dominant, and O recessive.

Statistical investigation of ABO blood groups across the world shows a high frequency of O in northwest Europe, southwest Africa, parts of Australia, and among the Indians of central and south America. Frequency of A is high in Europe and western Asia, and among Australian aborigines; while B is less frequent in Europe but reaches high frequency in central Asia and northern India. In both the USA and Britain the relative frequency of the groups is about the same: O, 45%; A, 41-43 %; B, 9-10%; AB, 3-4%. Over the years, more divisions of blood type (called grouping systems) have been discovered, for example, Rhesus, MN, AK, PGM, etc. As more and more statistical information becomes available on the frequency of occurrence of these systems in different groups of the world population, it becomes increasingly possible that a forensic scientist, given a specimen of unidentified blood, may be able to determine the ethnic group from which it is derived.

Work in the average forensic science laboratory begins with tests to discover whether or not the sample is blood, and then whether it is human or not. Usually a small piece of stained clothing is clipped out, while stains on wood, plaster or metal are usually scraped into a watch glass, though sometimes, as in the Thompsen case, whole sections of woodwork or plaster may be removed for thorough testing. As a general rule, the more recent the bloodstain, the greater its solubility. Stains on fabrics which have subsequently been washed or ironed are less soluble — a fact which may often have a bearing on the case in question, for obvious reasons.

The preliminary tests for blood are devoted to detecting the presence of an enzyme that releases oxygen from hydrogen peroxide. A preliminary test for blood is the Kastle-Meyer test. A piece of dry filter paper is rubbed on to the stain so that some of the stain is transferred on to the paper. Reagents (alcohol, phenolphthalein solution and hydrogen peroxide) are added dropwise and in order to the filter paper. The formation of a pinkish coloration is positive, and will reveal the presence of blood in extremely low concentrations. Further confirmation may be obtained by spectroscopic analysis.

Criminals, of course, frequently try to remove bloodstains from various materials, but they are seldom entirely successful. Bleach, for instance, will turn the colouring matter of blood to a greenish-brown. There is nothing more successful than prolonged soaking in water, although this will not remove all the blood. In one case, blood was detected, 60 days after the crime, in shoes that had been washed and then regularly worn.

The next stage is to determine whether the blood is human or animal, and this is achieved by using an antiserum which will react specifically with human blood. Once the presence of human blood is established, the complicated procedure of classifying blood groups begins.

At the moment, as mentioned earlier, it is usually impossible to state that a particular bloodstain definitely came from a particular person, but it is possible to conclude that a bloodstain did not come from a given source. In the past few years rapid strides have been taken in the direction of using blood samples as a means of positive identification; it has been discovered that the frequencies of the various genes within different blood group systems vary from race to race and could possibly provide important evidence.

In most cases it is already possible to tell the 'sex' of a blood-stain, as the white corpuscles of females show minute drumstick-shaped marks when examined microscopically. An interesting case involving this factor occurred in Britain during the early seventies, when a man was alleged to have raped a girl. When the man was arrested, the girl indicated bloodstains on the lining of his mackintosh, where, she said, he had wiped his blood-stained penis. The man denied the assault, and claimed that the blood on the raincoat was his own. A forensic serologist asked for samples from both the accused and the alleged victim, and both volunteered. Unfortunately, their blood groups were proved to be identical. Nevertheless the scientist examined the stains on the mackintosh, and found them to be female. The man was convicted.

At the Home Office central research establishment, Aldermaston, scientists have already revealed new directions in blood identification, and claim hopefully that one day they may be able to detail a criminal's age, sex, travelling habits, and diet from a sample of his blood. For instance, age can already be guessed roughly, for the antibodies, the natural protection against disease, build up through life and then gradually disappear, so that the very young and the very old have 'low disease profiles'.

They also know that antibodies from common allergies build up differently in the blood depending on the area in which the allergy is contracted; in America, for instance, hay fever is caused by rag-weed, while in Britain it comes from a different grass.

Already, since the 1950s, acid phosphatase has been used as a test for the presence of semen in cases of alleged rape – although, of course, semen may not be present, as ejaculation by the male is not necessary for rape to have taken place. In the routine 'AP reaction' test, as it is known, a chemical is broken down in a complex chemical procedure and a test solution produced which, if semen is present, exhibits a bright purple colour. A 'quick test' for possible seminal staining has been in use since the 1920s, and involves subjecting the undergarments of both accused and accuser to the light of a filtered ultraviolet lamp. However, stains caused by urine, vaginal discharge and other substances may also show as whitish fluorescence, therefore this test is not conclusive.

Semen is as amenable to 'grouping' as blood, and its analysis is an important factor not only in cases of criminal assault but also in questions of paternity. When a rape is alleged to have taken place, the medical examiner will take swabs from the vagina – in the case of rape and murder he also takes anal and oral swabs – to test for the presence of semen. These can be matched, or otherwise, against the suspect's semen. In fact, semen tests in sexual charges have been going on for a surprisingly long time, as Dr Alfred Swaine Taylor, one of the fathers of British forensic research, reported in the 1840s.

The case came before the Edinburgh courts on 27 November 1843. Dr Taylor reported:

A man labouring at that time under gonorrhoea was charged with a criminal assault on a child. The shift worn by the prosecutrix, with other articles belonging to the prisoner, were submitted for examination. Some of the stains on the linen were of a yellow colour, and were believed to be those of gonorrhoea; others, characterized by a faint colour and peculiar odour, were considered to be stains caused by the spermatic secretion. Digested in water, they yielded a turbid solution of a peculiar odour, and when submitted to a powerful microscope, spermatozoa were detected. The stains were similar on the linen of the prisoner and the prosecutrix. I believe this to be a solitary instance of the use of the microscope for such a purpose in this country.

Closely allied to serology in crime investigation is the study of hair and fibres. Flimsy though it may seem, human hair, unless burned or treated with acid, is virtually indestructible and is often found adhering to the skeletons of long buried bodies. It retains arsenic and certain other poisons more or less indefinitely, and although a single hair is a less positive clue than, for instance, a portion of fingerprint or even a smear of blood, it may occasionally prove of value to forensic scientists. Microscopic examination can sometimes provide indications of the age, sex and race of a hair owner, and can link a suspect to a crime scene, or a victim to a weapon.

The three obvious characteristics of hair found at the scene of a crime are length, colour, and texture, but when placed under a powerful microscope an individual hair will reveal a variety of further useful properties. A single hair is made up of three portions. The core or medulla, which is surrounded by the cortex, made up of a horny substance called keratin, and the outer layer or cuticle, which is composed of tiny overlapping scales. The scales of the cuticle play a vital part in matching and identifying hairs as they vary from animal to animal. An expert can rapidly distinguish an animal from a human hair, and can usually tell from what type of creature the hair came. Dog or cat hairs found on a suspect may place him at the scene of a crime, for instance.

The part of the body from which a hair has originated is also distinguished. Head hairs are usually circular in section, and if they have been neglected tend to 'split' at the ends. Freshly cut hair is square at the end and to a certain extent the time between haircuts can be established by its growth.

Eyebrow hairs are similar in section to head hairs but taper at the ends, while hairs from the beard and moustache – which may also show signs of trimming – may be triangular in section. Body and pubic hairs are oval or triangular and tend to curl in most individuals. More importantly, pubic hairs are less deeply rooted than head hairs, and are usually to be found after a sexual attack: along with seminal stains they are among the first signs rape investigators look for. The usual signs watched for are those of lacquering, tinting, dyeing or artificial curling, and an examination of the chemicals used in hair treatment can be of assistance.

For examination in the crime laboratory, hair is usually

mounted on a glass slide for viewing on a comparison microscope. For viewing in cross section, a sample is embedded in a wax or resin block and sliced finely, after which the cross section and the appearance of the medulla can be microscopically examined, while impressions of the cuticle scales are made on cellulose acetate for careful study.

A great deal was made of 'hair' evidence by the press at the time of the murder of Vivian Messiter in 1928. Sir Bernard Spilsbury found two eyebrow hairs on the murder weapon, a pointed ended hammer, which matched a wound over the victim Messiter's left eye. At the time of the trial a newspaper announced: 'Two hairs hanged this man!', going on to speak of the 'most vital clue of all'.

As Spilsbury was quick to point out, the evidence of the hair merely established that the hammer had been used in the slaying; it was dogged police work and the activities of another branch of the forensic laboratory which finally brought the killer to justice, an example of the evaluation which each forensic investigator must put on the pieces of evidence he brings to bear.

Typically, it was Sir Sydney Smith who perhaps pieced together the most classic case in which blood, semen – or its absence – and hair evidence solved a tragic case which dominated the headlines of both the British and overseas press in the 1930s.

At half past one on the afternoon of 20 April 1934, an eight-year-old girl named Helen Priestly was sent by her mother to buy bread at a store a few minutes' walk away from their tenement home in Aberdeen. Helen was a punctual child, and when she had not reappeared after some time, Mrs Priestly went out to look for her. The assistants at the shop said she had bought the bread and taken it away with the voucher slip recording the sale just after half past one. Mrs Priestly began to scour the area, and as the afternoon wore on and the news came that the girl had not turned up for school she called her husband home and told the police.

The tenement dwellers, who lived on four floors, with two flats to each floor, were a neighbourly people, and when they heard of Helen's disappearance they turned out to help in the search: all, that is, except Alexander and Jeannie Donald, who lived in the flat below the Priestlys, and with whom Mrs Priestly was not on speaking terms. The search went on all night, until at five in the morning a neighbour named William Topp found Helen's body near a water closet on the ground floor of the tenement. What puzzled Topp, and the police, was that he had used the water closet on that floor earlier in the night and swore that the body had not been there at the time.

Dr Richards, police surgeon for the city of Aberdeen, was called. The body, he discovered, was lying in a sack, fully clothed except for knickers and beret. The imprint of the store voucher was on the palm of her hand, but there was no sign of the bread. The sack also contained some cinders, some of which had lodged in her hair and her mouth, and she had vomited on her dress. The body was lying on its right side, but post-mortem lividity showed that it had lain on its left for several hours after death.

Rigor mortis had set in, there was blood on her thighs and dress, and she had suffered very serious injuries to her private parts. Because of this, and because the body had obviously been placed by someone who had ready access to the tenements, the police began questioning all the men in the eight flats which made up the building. Meanwhile, Dr Roberts and Professor Shennan, Professor of Pathology at Aberdeen University had begun work on the autopsy.

The outer skin of the neck showed signs of strangulation, and when the body was opened vomited matter was found in the windpipe and the smaller air tubes, while bruises, typical of manual strangulation, were found on the voice box and windpipe. The two experts gave asphyxia from strangulation as the cause of death. An examination of the stomach revealed Helen's last meal of meat and potatoes, eaten at half past twelve, and the digestive changes showed that death had taken place not later than two in the afternoon.

As the police discovered, the male inhabitants of the tenement had firm alibis for this period, for they were all at work. This fact changed the course of the investigation when details of the autopsy became known, for despite the deep penetration and tearing of the child's sexual organs, no semen was present, and in fact closer examination showed that her injuries had probably been caused by a sharp stick of some kind. The conclusion drawn from this was that someone had tried to make the death look like rape – the injuries had been inflicted before death – and it seemed reasonable to suppose that a woman would be more likely to do this, in order to divert attention. Two more pieces of evidence came to light; Helen had been seen walking towards her home at about 1.45 pm., and had apparently entered the tenement – passing the Donald's door as she did so. Further, a slater working on a nearby roof reported having heard a child's scream at about 2 pm.

As a matter of routine the police questioned the Donalds, along with the other families. Mrs Donald admitted that she and her husband had been the only ones not to help in the search, and that there was bad blood between her and the Priestlys. She gave what appeared at first to be a clear account of her movements on the afternoon of the murder – she had been out shopping between about 1.10 and 2.15, and had come back to see Mrs Priestly sobbing on the street corner, surrounded by friends. She had then gone in and spent the afternoon ironing. However, certain parts of her story did not stand up – a shop that she claimed to have visited had been closed all day on the Friday for one thing – and after the police found what appeared to be a bloodstain in her house, Mrs Donald, along with her husband, was arrested. As it chanced the stain turned out not to be blood at all, but the police were by now strongly suspicious. Although Alexander Donald's alibi proved firm and he was released, Mrs Donald remained in her cell. At this point Smith was called in, as conviction, it appeared, could only be achieved by means of medical and scientific evidence.

He saw immediately that two lines of investigation were open; one was to look for items found on the body of the girl which could be identified with the Donald household, and the other was to check for clues which may have been overlooked if and when the Donalds had cleaned up after the killing.

Examining the sack, Smith found that it was of a Canadian make, used to ship cereals to Aberdeen. Mr Donald's brother had been in the habit of bringing back potatoes in similar sacks, but this was not strong evidence. However, five similar sacks were found in the flat, and all of them had holes in one corner where they had hung from a hook – as had the 'murder' sack.

Inside the death sack, Smith found the cinders and a small amount of household fluff, containing a few human and animal hairs. Checking out the cinders he found only one thing of significance – they had been washed, a habit which only Mrs Donald out of the whole tenement block had. But the hairs were of far greater interest. Firstly, they were not those of the child. They were of a different colour and much coarser.

They showed a remarkable irregularity of contour and had many defined twists. This peculiarity was caused by rather careless artificial waving. Hair that we obtained from a brush supplied to Mrs Donald while she was in prison showed exactly similar characteristics and a similar waving distortion. As far as I could judge by examination in a comparison microscope, the hairs from the sack and those from Mrs Donald were identical in every detail.

Unfortunately, even this was not clinching evidence. Smith set to work on the rest of the fluff, and found traces of cat and rabbit hair, along with fibres of wool, cotton, silk, linen and jute dyed different colours – over two hundred different fibres in all. These were compared with similar samples taken from the Donald household under the comparison microscope and also using microchemical and spectroscopic tests. No fewer than 25 different fibres were matched, including the human and animal hair. Examples of fluff were taken from the other houses in the tenement, and in no case was a single match produced.

The instrument used to injure Helen was never found, nor were her beret or knickers, but a loaf of bread similar to that which she had bought was discovered – it was of a type not normally eaten by the Donalds – and in the fireplace a burned scrap of paper appeared to be the voucher she had carried, though this could not be proved absolutely.

Bloodstains were found on various items in the flat; on two washing cloths, a scrubbing brush, a packet of soap flakes, a piece of linoleum and two newspapers dated the day before the crime. The child's blood group was shown to be group O, as were the stains on the objects found. The defence refused permission to group Mrs Donald's blood, but with typical resource Smith obtained one of her used sanitary towels from the prison, and discovered that her blood was of a different type altogether.

Again this was only circumstantial evidence, for group O is common and in those days testing techniques were not as sophisticated as today; nevertheless a damning picture was building up.

Professor Smith was far from finished with his blood testing, in any case, and it was probably his next deduction which clinched matters. Examining the girl's wounds afresh, he realized that her blood may have been contaminated by bacteria as a result of a rupture of the intestinal canal; therefore he sent her bloodstained clothing, together with certain bloodstained articles from the Donald household, to be examined at the University's Department of Bacteriology.

The germs found in the child's combinations differed in certain respects from the ordinary intestinal bacteria. The bacterial strains from one of the washing cloths . . . showed a close similarity to the more unusual strains derived from the child's combinations. By tests of a highly technical nature a definite relationship was established between the strain from the cloth and the strain from the child.

The trial of Jeannie Donald began on 16 July 1934. A hundred and sixty four witnesses, many of them experts who had helped Professor Smith, were called, and he produced 253 separate items for the prosecution's case. Even the counsel for the defence described the Professor's efforts as 'careful and meticulous preparation unparalleled in the history of this old court'.

The 'old court' was, in fact, the Edinburgh High Court, for considerable public prejudice had built up against the Donalds, and the trial lasted five days, much of this time, of course, being taken up with medical and scientific evidence. None of the laboratory findings were conclusive in themselves, but the sum total made a strong case. Smith's theory of method and motive was that Helen had made some sort of objectionable remark to Mrs Donald as she passed her door, and that Mrs Donald caught her shoulder and shook her. At the post-mortem, it had been discovered that Helen suffered from an overgrowth of lymphatic tissue; a child with this condition is liable to lose consciousness extremely rapidly and unexpectedly, and it was possible that Mrs Donald thought the child had died. Pulling her into the house, she thought frantically and decided to simulate rape with the sharp instrument; the pain awoke Helen and she screamed and vomited, swallowing some of the vomit. This may have been the cause of death, though the bruises suggested that Jeannie Donald had strangled her to be sure. Then she had stuffed the body into a sack, possibly putting in the cinders in order to soak up the blood, and had awaited her opportunity to dispose of the body in the dead of night, while the other occupants of the building were out searching. She then washed up throughly, only neglecting to wash the cloths properly afterwards. 'In one of those cloths,' as Smith said, 'was the immensely important bacterial strain.'

The jury took only 18 minutes to find Jeannie Donald guilty, and she was sentenced to death, afterwards commuted to life imprisonment partly because of the plea of the humane Smith, who felt that she had no deliberate intent to kill the child.

The one point of humour in the whole dreadful tragedy was pinpointed by Smith years later. The trial cost an estimated £3,000, 'and', he commented, 'I believe that the change of venue [to Edinburgh] was greatly appreciated by the thrifty citizens of Aberdeen, since the expenses in the High Court would be met by the Crown, and not fall on the Aberdeen rates'.

# Chapter Eleven
# With poison deadly

The strongest poison ever known
Came from Caesar's laurel crown.

William Blake, *Auguries of Innocence*

Homicidal poisoning has always presented medico-legal examiners with something of a paradox. The first relatively detailed
accounts of it occur in the records of the Roman Empire around
the time of Christ, but by then it was already an ancient art for
the Egyptians, and before them the Chinese, who had practised
it for centuries as a sophisticated way of killing.

In modern statistical terms poisoning comes low on the
murder index; in an average year in the United States, 51
percent of homicides are committed with handguns, 20 percent
with knives or other stabbing and cutting weapons, 9 percent
are committed through purely personal violence – strangling,
kicking, and so on – while shotguns and rifles account for 8 and
6 percent respectively. Of the remaining six percent, which
includes such relatively esoteric crimes as running down with
automobiles, euthanasia, and the like, deliberate poisoning
takes up no more than half.

Most criminologists agree on the rarity of poison as a murder
weapon. Professor Keith Simpson put it succinctly, 'Homicide
by poison is rare', he wrote. 'The Maybricks, Seddons, Crippens
and Merryfields are famous only because they are of rare
interest.' Crime writer Colin Wilson makes another point:

In real life – as in fiction – it is always easier to identify and bring a
poisoner to trial than it is to get the bandit before the jury for the
dollars stolen from a bank. Poisoning is usually a personal affair, with
a motive like a shining beacon. This is why the clear-up rate for
poisoners . . . is far higher than with any other type of crime.

But there is another side to the matter. The apparent rarity of
poisoning as a crime may be due to the fact that many cases go
undetected, particularly with the increasing use of, for instance,

barbiturates in suicide attempts, and in cases where the symptoms can superficially be attributed to natural causes. A leading toxicologist commented:

I have seen cases in which the family doctor has registered cause of death as food poisoning or the like, and I've performed an autopsy as a matter of course and found that poison has been administered deliberately. Granted, most of these cases involve suicidal attempts, but one wonders how many general practitioners would recognise a case of homicidal arsenic poisoning today. Its very rarity means that the average busy medical man isn't going to be looking for it.

Indeed, the materials at the disposal of a would-be poisoner are formidable: the 1946 edition of Glaister's *Medical Jurisprudence* – published before the widespread use of barbiturates – lists around five hundred possible causes of death by poisoning, ranging from absinthe through to weever fish stings, and many of them have alarmingly similar symptoms. And despite the rigid controls practised in the Western world where all drugs are concerned, each new synthetic drug presents potential to a killer. Indeed, each advance in medical science has its dark side, typified, perhaps, by the unsuccessful attempt, in the spring of 1978, of a German laboratory technician to kill his wife by administering cancer cells to her. He worked in a cancer research centre, managed to smuggle out a cancer culture, and mixed it with his wife's food. In fact, although she became sick, she did not die, since that culture was not in itself dangerous in this form. Similarly, the scare which followed the discovery that a large consignment of oranges from Israel had been injected with metallic mercury was without foundation, although the fruit was withdrawn from the market. Mercury in a metallic state is relatively innocuous – indeed it was taken orally as a treatment for syphilis in the eighteenth century – and it is only when injected into the veins or inhaled in a dust or vapour state that it becomes toxic.

Because of the complex nature of poisons, and the fact that their effects may be misunderstood by those administering them, the present law of Great Britain – though not of the United States – contains an 'escape clause' with regard to poisoners or potential poisoners. The Offences Against the

Person Act states that it is a felony to 'administer or cause to be administered' poisons with intent to commit murder, but in some cases modern prosecuting counsel will accept a 'not guilty' plea of 'intent to cause grievous bodily harm' and substitute the lesser charge of 'administering poison with the intent of injuring, grieving or annoying'.

Due to this clause an 18-year-old boy from Manchester, England, walked from the local Crown Court to freedom, despite having told the judge of a silly prank which could have killed the entire staff of the factory in which he worked. In July 1973 the boy was prosecuted for malicious poisoning, and the court heard how he had poured cyanide into the milk used for making tea in the factory canteen. He had intended to 'upset' the woman in charge of his section, and a 17-year-old workmate against whom he bore a grudge. Fortunately just before the morning tea break a canteen assistant poured a saucer of the milk for two kittens, which promptly went into convulsions and died. Enquiries were made, the police called, and the boy arrested.

The judge, Sir William Morris, gave the boy a six-month prison sentence, suspended for two years, and told him: 'It was a wicked thing you did, and you might have been standing here on a very serious charge of killing.'

Some poisoners have been known to use the solid cyanide used as rat poison and insecticide, though photographic laboratories, plating works and process engraving plants use the commercially pure potassium cyanide; although there are tight controls in its industrial use, poisoning by potassium cyanide may not create immediate suspicion if it involves a worker in such an industry.

Curiously, though cyanide is often thought of, with arsenic, as one of the most sinister poisons, and although 300 milligrams constitute a lethal dose, it is not always a sure killer. When stored it tends to deteriorate, and quite a large amount can be taken without proving fatal, providing a doctor is called in time to rinse the stomach by tube and administer stimulants such as amyl nitrite and detoxicants like sodium thiosulphate.

One of the great cyanide poisoning mysteries of the twentieth century was probably solved, in retrospect, by Professor Keith Simpson: that involving the death of Grigori Rasputin, the 'mad monk' whose hold over the wife of Tsar Nicholas II made him virtual ruler of Russia in the years immediately preceding the revolution.

On the night of 29 December 1916, Prince Felix Yussopov and three like-minded friends decided to rid Russia of the peasant-born dictator. They invited Rasputin to a party at Yussopov's house, and the 'holy devil', as he was nicknamed went along gladly, apparently in the hope of seducing Princess Irina, Yussopov's wife, who was in fact away in the Crimea.

Arriving about midnight, he immediately fell upon the wine and chocolate cake provided for him by the Prince in a luxuriously furnished cellar apartment; the food and drink, as Yussopov later maintained, 'contained enough potassium cyanide to kill a monastery of monks'.

To the consternation of Yussopov and his companions, the monk drank glass after glass and ate mounds of the cake apparently quite happily. Finally the Prince shot him in the back at point blank range. Two hours later, however, Rasputin revived, hauled himself to his feet and ripped Yussopov's uniform. Two more bullets were fired at him, and he was battered around the head with a steel press before being pushed, still alive, beneath the frozen waters of the river Neva. Two days later his body was washed up, the right arm frozen in the act of making the sign of the cross.

When details of the killing, and the monk's remarkable staying power, leaked out, Yussopov's objective was all but lost; superstitious peasants whispered that Rasputin had indeed been a 'holy devil'.

Since then, forensic scientists and criminologists have debated the case, the details of which were unswervingly averred by Prince Yussopov, who died in Paris in the 1960s. The bullets Rasputin may well have survived; stranger cases have happened, and he had a giant constitution. The same applied to the battering, and the icy water of the river may actually have revived him. But what of the huge dose of poison?

Professor Keith Simpson has pointed out that cyanide is more or less harmless until it comes into contact with the gastric juices, so that its action in the body may be delayed by 'dyspepsia'. 'Should the victim suffer from chronic gastritis as Rasputin probably did', he wrote, 'he may swallow many times the fatal dose and escape the fate an ordinary subject would quickly meet.'

The misuse of drugs as alleged aphrodisiacs has frequently been the subject of criminal proceedings, where the defendant usually admits that he had no prior knowledge of the fatally toxic effect of the substance administered. Perhaps the most famous 'aphrodisiac' of folk lore is 'Spanish Fly' made from the dried beetle *Cantharis* (Lytta) *vesicatoria*, which is widely found in areas of southern Europe. The active ingredient of the prepared insect is cantharidin, and the powdered product contains around 0.6 percent of the substance. Sometimes a tincture of cantharidin is made, and the fatal dose is usually reckoned at 1.5 to 3 grams of the powder, or about 200 millilitres of the tincture.

In fact, cantharidin is a blistering agent, which irritates the mucous membranes not only of the vagina but also of the mouth, intestines and so on. In small doses it may well produce a 'sexual itch' but it is extremely dangerous, and can cause agonising death. In Spain, southern France and areas of Italy it is traditionally used also as an abortion agent, but again usually proves fatal in this respect not only to the foetus but to the mother. If a forensic examiner suspects cantharidin poisoning, he usually looks for remnants of the insect's wing case in the stomach contents.

One of the most sensational cases involving cantharidin came to London's Old Bailey in 1954, when a wholesale chemist's manager named Arthur Kendrick Ford was tried on charges of manslaughter involving two of the girls who worked for him, 27-year-old Betty Grant and June Malins, a 17-year-old beauty queen.

Ford, 44 years old and apparently happily married, had conceived a desire for both Miss Grant and Miss Malins, and remembered the rumours he had heard about the alleged aphrodisiac qualities of 'Spanish Fly' in the army. One day he discovered that the technical term for Spanish fly was cantharidin, and that supplies were available at his place of work. He asked the firm's senior chemist, Mr Richard Lushington, if he could obtain some cantharidin because, said Ford, one of his neighbours was breeding rabbits and he felt that cantharidin might play 'a useful part in the mating process'.

Mr Lushington told him that the drug was a 'number one poison' and, if administered to a human being in anything in excess of half a milligram, could be fatal. Nevertheless he gave Ford – a man of previously unimpeachable character – a small quantity of the drug. Ford, who was a friendly and popular man, went out on 26 April 1954, and bought a bag of pink and white coconut ice candy. Back in the office, he admitted, he pushed quantities of the cantharidin into the candy with a pair of scissors, and gave a piece to Miss Grant, and a piece to Miss Malin, and ate a piece himself.

Within an hour all three were sick, and were taken to University College Hospital nearby. The next day the two girls died but Ford, though violently ill, survived. University College is a major hospital with a highly trained staff of toxicologists; the post-mortems on the two girls quickly revealed the presence of cantharidin in their bodies – their internal organs had been 'literally burned away by the drug' according to evidence.

Interviewed by police, Ford echoed the cry of most 'accidental' poisoners: 'Oh dear God what an awful thing I have done!' he said. 'Why didn't somebody tell me? I have been an awful fool.' For his folly he was sentenced to five years imprisonment.

It has recently been suggested that an accident of exactly the opposite kind to that which resulted in the Ford tragedy may have played a part in one of the most famous poisoning cases of all time – the Crippen episode. Harvey Hawley Crippen, though not licensed to practise medicine in Britain, nevertheless had respectable American medical qualifications. In London, where his wife Cora wanted desperately to establish herself as a vaudeville star, he became a herbalist and pedlar of 'quack' medicines – or so his detractors over the years have claimed. The fact is that he was probably as competent a pharmacologist as most doctors of medicine.

Crippen seems to have sacrificed a great deal to his wife's ambition, including his own legitimate career in accompanying her to England. She repaid him by openly flaunting her sexual charms and was almost certainly unfaithful to him with men friends in the theatre – she was a boon companion of Marie Lloyd, whose own appetite for men was notorious. Shortly before she disappeared, Dr Crippen purchased 5 grains (300 milligrams) of the vegetable drug hyoscine hydrobromide (now used in treatment of motion sickness) from a shop in Oxford Street – it was such a large dose that it had to be specially obtained from the wholesalers. From his work in the United States with psychiatric patients, Crippen knew that the drug was a powerful anaphrodisiac – it dampened the sexual ardours of those who took it. It has been suggested that perhaps the little doctor bought the drug for precisely this purpose: to stop Cora's philanderings; and that instead he accidentally killed her. About 217 milligrams of hyoscine hydrobromide were found in her remains, and as he appears to have been the first recorded murderer in history to use the drug, it seems unlikely that he knew precisely what a fatal dose constituted.

Doctors, because of their ready access to dangerous drugs, constitute a large section of those poisoners known to criminal historians. Most 'killer doctors' have used such drugs as morphine or its derivatives in their crimes – drugs which are usually legitimately carried in their bags.

Morphine is the most powerful of the opiate groups of drugs, which all stem from the dried juice of the white Indian poppy, *Papaver somniferum*. All of the plant's products are narcotics – they reduce pain and induce semi or total unconsciousness – and all are habit-forming.

In Victorian times, before drugs were brought under control, laudanum, or tincture of opium – which contains 1 percent morphine – was widely used as an opiate; such writers as Thomas De Quincy, who wrote *Memoirs of an Opium Eater*, and Patrick Branwell Brontë, brother of the three famous Brontë sisters, became addicts. Other products such as paregoric or chlorodyne contain varying amounts of morphine and may cause death by overdose.

In many wars since the early nineteenth century, doctors on the world's battlefields have used morphine as a handy painkiller – it can be administered either orally or by injection – though the effects were in many cases disastrous, for the drug is highly addictive, and patients rapidly acquire a 'tolerance' for it. The normal dose of hydromorphine hydrochloride is 2 milligrams, but addicts have been known to take up to 900 times this amount – thirty times the toxic dose.

Morphine deaths are usually accompanied by deep, slow respiration, coma, and profuse sweating; but besides these signs the forensic expert will usually spot morphine poisoning because of the pinpoint contraction of the pupils which accompanies it.

Where morphine death is suspected, containers at the scene are tested for the drug; morphine in its ordinary state turns a bluish colour when treated with ferric chloride and an instant purple, in its dry state, when touched with a solution of concentrated sulphuric acid and formaldehyde. After a post-mortem, the blood, urine and bile are checked chemically for morphine traces.

In May 1947, a Doctor Robert Clements called another doctor to his Southport, Cheshire, home to attend his fourth wife, who was in a deep coma. The 57-year-old doctor told his colleague that Mrs Clements was suffering from myeloid leukaemia, and when she died the following morning the disease was entered on her certificate as the cause of death. Two doctors, Brown and Homes, were slightly unhappy about the situation, however, for they spotted that Mrs Clements's eyes had retracted into the typical 'pin-point' state associated with morphine poisoning. A third medical man, Dr Houston, performed an autopsy and pronounced that the cause of death was indeed leukaemia. Nevertheless Brown and Homes were so disturbed that they reported their suspicions to the coroner.

When the police began their enquiries they discovered that a number of acquaintances of the Clements had noted that things did not seem quite right with the couple. Mrs Clements, for instance, was subject to sudden bouts of unconsciousness, though her husband always seemed to know when they would occur. He had also recently had the telephone removed from their home – an odd action for a busy doctor with a sick wife. Her health had deteriorated over a period of time; she had vomited regularly, her complexion had turned yellowish, and she was lethargic – all signs of morphine overdosing. Then it was discovered that Dr Clements had prescribed a huge dose of morphine for a non-existent patient, and a second autopsy was ordered. The Home Office pathologist found that the body was incomplete; certain organs, he discovered, had been destroyed by order of Dr Houston after the first autopsy. Nonetheless he decided that Mrs Clements had in fact died of morphine poisoning, and the police called upon Dr Clements. They found him dead – of morphine poisoning. In a suicide note he had written that he could 'no longer tolerate the diabolical insults to which I have recently been exposed'.

The police then hastened to Dr Houston's surgery, and found that he too had taken his own life, this time with cyanide. He had left a note confessing that he had made 'mistakes' in his work.

The coroner's court found Clements guilty of killing his fourth wife, who had been the heiress of a large fortune which he would have inherited had all gone as he had apparently planned. Enquiries also showed that all his three previous wives had been wealthy. Furthermore all died of illnesses 'diagnosed' by the doctor himself, and he had signed all their death certificates.

If Clements had read of the Buchanan case of 1892 he might have made at least an attempt to cover up his tracks. Dr Robert Buchanan, a Scottish-American, had qualified at Edinburgh, married, and returned to New York in 1886, where he set up practice. By day he was a respected medical man, but by night he took to frequenting brothels and low-life clubs. In November 1890 he divorced his wife and married Anna Sutherland, a rich brothel madame who shortly afterwards changed her will in his favour.

Unfortunately, his new wife refused to give up her lucrative if seamy business, and she quickly became a liability to Buchanan, who was by this time amassing a roster of well-to-do patients. On 25 April 1892, he announced that he was returning to Edinburgh to further his medical studies, leaving his wife behind. Anna, however, announced that she would either accompany him or she would cut him out of her will. Buchanan cancelled his passage, and a few days afterward announced that his wife had become seriously ill.

Some time later she died, and the cause of death was certified as brain haemorrhage: Buchanan inherited $50,000. Anna's former partner was dissatisfied with the result of the autopsy and went to the police to complain of Buchanan. They refused to take action on the word of a pimp against such a notable figure but the *New York World* thought otherwise. Its reporters began asking questions, and soon discovered that Dr Buchanan had secretly remarried his first wife only 23 days after Anna's death. The medical examiner who had performed the post-mortem examination, however, flatly refused to consider the suggestion that Mrs Buchanan had died of anything other than brain haemorrhage. The reporters reminded him of another New York case in 1891 where a medical student named Harris had poisoned his wife with morphine and the death had at first been taken for cerebral haemorrhage.

The medical examiner pointed out that in the Harris case, pin-pointing of the pupils had been present. There was no such symptom in the case of Anna Buchanan. Nevertheless, the *New York World* pressured the New York coroner, through its columns, for a fresh investigation, and an exhumation order was granted. Professor Witthaus, an eminent toxicologist, found that the body contained 1/10th of a grain of morphine in the remains, which he estimated was the residue of a fatal dose of 2 or 3 grains (150-200 milligrams). On this evidence Dr Buchanan was placed on trial in March 1893.

Witnesses for the prosecution claimed that they had heard Dr Buchanan, at the time of the Harris case, refer to the accused as a 'bungling fool' and a 'stupid amateur'. He had claimed that a few drops of belladonna in the eyes of the victim would permanently halt the tell-tale 'pin-point' symptoms; in court a nurse who had attended Mrs Buchanan confirmed that the doctor had put drops in his wife's eyes for no apparent reason. The prosecution conducted a bizarre experiment in which they actually killed a cat, in court, with morphine, and put belladonna in its eyes, thus stopping the pin-point process. In turn the defence showed that the colour reaction tests used by Dr Witthaus to identify the presence of morphine were not infallible. But with the defence swinging the case in his favour, Dr Buchanan arrogantly elected to enter the witness box in his own defence, and was quickly torn to pieces by the district attorney. He was found guilty of murder and electrocuted at Sing Sing in July 1895.

Modern toxicological methods are fortunately much more precise than those available to Dr Buchanan's prosecutors, and such a ruse as his in using the belladonna drops would not go undetected for long in a modern laboratory. Furthermore such modern methods as colour reactions (updated from those used by Dr Witthaus), thin-layer chromatography, and gas chromatography can identify the presence of most poisons down to amounts as small as 1/5000th of a grain.

As an American toxicologist rather flamboyantly put it:

The 'Big M' can brand a man, and may stand for mercy, misery or murder. But where homicides by morphine and the other opium derivatives are detected today, they generally tend to be caused by the dead person himself – suicidally or through an overdose. A modern doctor who wished to use morphine for murderous purposes would have to be an expert – much more skilled and much more wily in his methods than Dr Buchanan.

Professor Glaister, as late as the eighth edition of his *Medical Jurisprudence* (1945), was able to comment that 'arsenious acid, arsenious oxide, or white arsenic is the substance most commonly employed in homicidal poisoning'. That this is no longer true is largely due to the rigid drug controls introduced over the past decades, although the substance is still widely used in such industries as dyeing, papermaking, and taxidermy; certain weed killers contain arsenic in the form of a soluble sodium arsenite, but again the sale of such preparations is tightly restricted today.

But the fact of arsenic's ubiquity as a murderous poison even in the days when it was fairly readily accessible has always puzzled criminologists; certainly no knowledgeable murderer would normally employ the substance, for it has probably more 'built in' drawbacks as a weapon of homicide than any other drug. To begin with, once arsenic poisoning is suspected it is rapidly detected in the system. Since the mid-nineteenth century, such methods as the Marsh, Reinsch, and Gutzeit tests have detected even minute traces in the body tissues, so that once suspicion has fallen upon him the murderer has a slender chance of his crime going undetected.

Then there is the problem of administration. Arsenious oxide is practically insoluble in cold water, which will only dissolve between $\frac{1}{2}$ to 1 grain per ounce. In boiling liquids, up to 55 grains per ounce will be held in solution for as long as the water remains hot, but once it has cooled only 12 grains remain dissolved, while the remainder fall to the bottom of the vessel, leaving a whitish film. Glaister showed that 100 grains of arsenious oxide mixed with two teaspoonsfuls of cocoa, milk, and boiling water in a cup could not be detected either by appearance, taste or smell, but that when the drink cooled the milk curdled and the arsenic sedimented. Similar results are obtained with arrowroot, gruel and soup preparations.

Even should the intended victim fail to notice the startling change in his drink or soup, the suspended 12 grains is by no means a sure killer. Although the lowest recorded dosage causing death is 2 grains, much larger doses have been taken without fatal effect, and Glaister records a case of a woman who took 230 grains in a suicide attempt and after an uncomfortable three days made a complete recovery. Concentrated lethal doses have been administered in powder form, mixed with jam or chocolate cake, for instance, and it is possible for arsenic to be effective when injected into the body by rectal enema or vaginal douche, but for obvious reasons the last two methods are improbable where homicide is concerned.

Where death by acute arsenical poisoning has occurred, medical examiners generally treat the case as suicide or possibly accident rather than murder, if only because one huge lethal dose of the substance is instantly detectable to the person taking it. Time of death is usually estimated at between 12 and 36 hours although, as with many poisons, this factor is extremely variable, depending on the age, general condition, and size of the victim. The symptoms are violent and unpleasant; nausea, faintness and a burning pain in the stomach and intestines followed by continuous vomiting and diarrhoea, with blood and bile being passed, and eventual convulsions, coma, and death – often caused suddenly by cardiac failure.

In chronic arsenic poisoning – the administration of small

doses over a period of time which is the usual method of arsenic slayers – the symptoms are similar but less intense; they are accompanied by loss of body weight, hair loss, and intense thirst – which also occurs in acute poisoning and only increases the nausea. The eyes are watery, the tongue thick and coated, and eczema-like eruptions appear on the skin, which often takes on a yellowish jaundiced look. All these symptoms could be attributed, by a careless doctor, to other causes – food poisoning, for instance or, in the case of a known heavy drinker, the terminal effects of alcoholic poisoning, for arsenic affects the liver and kidneys. But any thorough examination of the patient should reveal arsenic poisoning.

The final drawback of an arsenic killer is the preservative powers of the substance. In large doses the poison remains in the body tissues, particularly the hair, fingernails and bones. Once there, it cannot be totally removed, even with powerful cleansing solutions. Furthermore the tissues tell a vital tale to the medico-legal examiner; hair and nails grow at a constant rate, and arsenic infiltrates them in a similarly constant manner, so that tests on a length of hair will show clearly when the poisoning began, when the last dose was taken and so on.

In some cases of murder by arsenic, the defence has argued, quite rightly, that most human bodies contain a small quantity of arsenic – although it is not a natural component of the body. It may be ingested in minute quantities through the use of certain soaps, by exposure to weed killer, or even, in gardeners, through contact with ordinary soil, for earth contains arsenic in differing quantities. For this reason, at an exhumation where arsenic is suspected, the pathologist is careful to take not only body samples but samples of earth from the grave, from the wood of the coffin, and from the shroud and coffin lining. Their content is compared with that of the body to ascertain whether or not the substance could have been absorbed into the corpse after burial.

Despite all these snags, it is usually admitted that numbers of arsenical poisoners have probably gone undetected. Undue arrogance, or impatience, or greed are the main factors which have undone the convicted arsenic killers; in every case they did not know where to stop, and drew suspicion upon themselves. It was greed, for instance, which brought Frederick Henry Seddon, a near neighbour and contemporary of Dr Crippen, to the gallows.

In July 1910, Miss Eliza Mary Barrow moved into Seddon's house at Tollington Park, North London, as a lodger, after quarrelling with her cousin, Mr Vonderahe, at whose home she had previously lived. She paid Seddon a rent of twelve shillings per week in the first few weeks of her stay, but when she confided her 'troubles' to him, the rent was abolished in a rather curious manner.

Seddon was an insurance assessor with some knowledge of financial matters. Miss Barrow told him that she possessed property worth about £4000 and that she had quarrelled with her relatives over this. Seddon sympathized and, using his glib powers of persuasion, convinced her that she would be better off were she to sign her India stock, worth £1600, to him in exchange for an annuity and the remission of her rent. By January 1911 Seddon's hold over her had increased to such an extent that she had signed some leasehold property she owned over to him, in exchange for his increasing her annuity to £3 per week. According to her cousin she always kept £400 in cash with her, and in June 1911 she drew out the remains of her capital from the bank, a total of £200. This meant that the complete capital of £4000 was either in Seddon's hands or on his premises.

In late August, Seddon's daughter Maggie went to a chemist's shop on nearby Crouch Hill and bought a threepenny packet of fly papers which contained arsenic and were clearly marked 'Poison'. On 1 September, Miss Barrow became seriously ill with vomiting and diarrhoea, and Seddon brought in his own medical practitioner, Dr Sworn, who diagnosed the case as 'epidemic diarrhoea', which was prevalent at the time. On 13 September she died, and after Dr Sworn had issued a death certificate stating the diarrhoea to be the cause of death she was buried in the same Finchley cemetery in which Cora Crippen had been interred almost a year previously.

It was some days after the funeral that Miss Barrow's cousin

Vonderahe heard of her death and went to see Seddon. He knew, he said, that his cousin had kept £400 or so in cash with her at all times, and he also knew that she had recently withdrawn £200 from the bank. Where was the money? Seddon said he had no idea. He found only £10 in her room when she died. Profoundly dissatisfied, Vonderahe went to the police, who began investigating Seddon's recent financial affairs. They discovered not only that Mrs Seddon had changed a number of five pound notes recently, but that Seddon himself had accepted a commission of twelve shillings and sixpence from the undertaker who buried Miss Barrow. Clever detection led them to the Crouch Hill chemist, who told them of the arsenic-impregnated fly papers bought by Seddon's daughter, and an autopsy was ordered. Sir William Willcox, senior analyst to the Home Office, discovered traces of arsenic in the liver and intestines to show that a dose of at least 5 grains of arsenic had been administered to the dead woman shortly before she died, and examination of the hair and teeth confirmed the presence of previous doses.

Confronted with this evidence, Seddon suggested that Miss Barrow had 'accidentally' drunk the water in which the arsenic impregnated fly papers had been placed; in fact the actual source of the arsenic used to kill the lodger was never satisfactorily explained. According to Willcox, however, the fly papers found on Seddon's premises contained a lethal dose, and Seddon was convicted and hanged. It seemed that Dr Sworn had been genuinely misled by Miss Barrow's symptoms, so that the death itself should have caused no suspicion. If Seddon had been satisfied with the property and stocks which he had obtained from his lodger in her lifetime, and had placated her cousin with at least part of the ready cash she was known to possess, he would probably have escaped detection. As it was, his greed proved his undoing.

There were many celebrated arsenic poisoning cases in the late nineteenth and early twentieth century, most of them following the familiar pattern: sudden death from 'stomach upset', suspicion aroused, exhumation of the corpse and the discovery of the killer drug, ending inevitably with the arrest of a relative, friend, or colleague of the victim. The longest lasting of such trials eventually resulted in an acquittal – largely as a result of disagreement between experts.

In July 1949, Marie Josephine Besnard was arrested in Loudun – the French provincial town which in the seventeenth century had become notorious for an outbreak of 'witchcraft' – on a charge of killing 13 people, including two husbands, her mother and her father-in-law, as well as various friends and acquaintances. The evidence which brought her to court followed the routine; her husband, Leon Besnard, had died in 1947 as a result of a heart attack, according to the death certificate. But an anonymous letter to the local public prosecutor caused an exhumation order to be issued, and a Dr Beraud discovered a large quantity of arsenic in the body. Enquiries were made, and charges of poisoning by arsenic were brought against her in respect of 12 other people.

Her first trial began in 1949, but it was not until 1961, after four appeals, that she was declared innocent on each indictment. The first doubts were sown when it was shown that Dr Beraud had sent jars containing portions of Marie's alleged victims for full analysis to the laboratory at Marseilles, but that in fact more jars than he had sent had arrived, and that some of these contained muscle, rather than intestinal tissue. This mix-up was never satisfactorily explained. Secondly, although Dr Beraud had said in a letter to the judge that he could distinguish 'by eye' the rings left in a test tube by an arsenical deposit, when handed several test tubes in court he was unable to do so. And a Professor Perperot gave expert evidence that any corpse dug up after a period of inhumation in the area around Marie's home town would contain enough arsenic to 'decimate a regiment of men – for the very good reason that the soil is steeped in arsenic'..

By the late fifties another team of toxicologists had been called in, and by using a Geiger counter had reaffirmed the presence of arsenic in the body samples. The results had been sent for checking to the British Atomic Authority, who found them to be 80 percent inaccurate.

At the final trial, in 1961, the last team of experts averred that the arsenic in the bodies tallied with the large amount of the substance in the soil around them. As the only 'positive' evidence against her was the scientific aspect, and as she had been brought to trial on the tittle tattle of her neighbours, Marie Besnard, who had become known as 'The Black Widow', was allowed to go free after an ordeal which had lasted 12 years.

Along with arsenic, strychnine was one of the most 'popular' homicidal poisons of the nineteenth century, though cases of murder by the drug are rare today, and it has always been impractical for 'personal' murders, for the symptoms are easily recognized and the chemical tests for its presence are among the most simple in toxicology.

Strychnine is an alkaloid extracted from the seeds of the tree *Strychnos nux-vomica* which grows in India and whose qualities were first reported in 1818. It has an exceptionally bitter taste, and is used in tonics and animal poisons. Whether given orally or by injection, strychnine enters the bloodstream rapidly and in medicinal doses, as part of such preparations as Tincture of Nux Vomica, affects the nervous system just enough to give a feeling of well-being; the senses are heightened and the mental processes become acute. Even as a tonic, however, its use is strictly controlled by the medical profession, and indeed it is never prescribed by American doctors.

One of the dangers of its medical use is that it comes out of solution in an alkaline mixture and accumulates at the bottom of the container, so that failure to shake the medicine properly has resulted in cases of overdosing.

Reaction to an overdose is swift and, depending on the state of the victim, can cause death almost immediately. The muscles twitch and breathing becomes laboured and the chest muscles begin to tighten, before the victim is seized by convulsions as the drug reaches the motor areas of the spinal chord. The back arches in a condition known as opisthotonos, leaving only the back of the head and the heels touching the surface on which the body lies, and forward or lateral arching of the body – emprosthotonos and pleurosthotonos – may also occur. Alterations to the face are as dramatic as those to the body; the face becomes dark and suffused because of breathing difficulties, and the mouth muscles produce a hideous grinning effect known as risus sardonicus, while the eyes are wild and staring, and the lower jaw sets rigidly.

Each spasm lasts between half a minute and two minutes, before the victim relaxes for a while. Then comes the next spasm. Because of the asphixiating qualities of the drug, death may occur during the first attack in persons who suffer from bronchitis or asthma, and suffocation is the usual cause of death, although exhaustion or heart failure may hasten the end.

Because of the clenching of the jaw, the onset of strychnine poisoning vaguely resembles the symptoms of tetanus or 'lock-jaw', but in the case of the former the lockjaw effect is only part of the general stiffening of the body muscles and does not pass off during the intervening periods of relaxation. As Glaister says: 'There is no other set of phenomena, from disease or poison, which is exactly comparable to that which follows the absorption of strychnine into the body.'

One hundred milligrams of strychnine taken orally is usually considered to constitute a fatal dose, but doses as low as 30 milligrams have resulted in death, and accidental handling of the drug has produced definite symptoms; Glaister records the case where a dose of 5 milligrams rubbed into the eye caused symptoms within four minutes. There are no typical post-mortem characteristics of strychnine poisoning, although the brain, lungs and spinal chord are usually congested. Analysis is usually made of urine, brain, and spinal cord. Suspected residues, usually colourless crystals, are treated with sulphuric acid and go into solution, and the edge of the solution is touched with a crystal of potassium chromate. Where strychnine is present the solution immediately turns purple and then crimson before fading completely.

For notorious 'mass' killers who struck down their victims haphazardly, the unique qualities of strychnine presented few problems except its particularly bitter taste, which had to be disguised. The mid-Victorian poisoner Dr William Palmer administered his fatal doses in brandy, while Doctor Thomas Neill Cream, who killed prostitutes in south and east London at the end of the nineteenth century and in fact claimed, falsely, on the gallows to be Jack the Ripper, gave his victims strychnine in ordinary medicines.

One 'personal' strychnine killing which might just have succeeded were it not – as in so many cases – for the vigilance of a local doctor, was the so-called 'Blue Anchor' murder of 1924. A French wireless mechanic named Jean-Pierre Vaquier fell in love with Mrs Poynter Jones, the wife of an English public house owner, while she was on holiday in France. In February 1924, he followed her back to England and put up at her husband Alfred's hotel, the 'Blue Anchor' in Byfleet, Surrey. There he continued his affairs with Mrs Jones, and the two of them enjoyed several drinking sessions with the husband, who was a near alcoholic.

Shortly after Vaquier's arrival in London, he visited Bland's chemists in Southampton Row and became friendly with the French-speaking pharmacist. Vaquier told him that his name was Vanker – which Bland subsequently spelled 'Wanker' in the poisons book – and that he was a well known wireless mechanic and inventor in France. He persuaded the reluctant Bland to sell him some strychnine for 'wireless experiments'.

Early in March Alfred Poynter Jones had a bad attack of influenza, which induced congestion in the lungs – he had a history of chest problems. Nevertheless he seemed to recover and carried on his drinking bouts as usual. One morning towards the end of March after a particularly heavy session, Jones came down into the inn parlour to take a dose of the 'bromo salts' which he always kept on the mantlepiece there. Watched by Vaquier, who sat in an armchair drinking coffee, he took a dose, and almost immediately began gasping for breath. His doctor, Carle, was called, but half an hour later Jones had died of suffocation. Although Dr Carle knew, of course, of Jones's chest complaint, he found the attack rather too sudden, particularly as he had examined his patient some days previously and found him to be clear. He ordered a post-mortem, and scraped up some crystals from the floor of the bar parlour. These, along with samples of the dead man's body fluids and tissues, he sent to the Home Office analyst, John Webster. Webster found that they contained strychnine, and Vaquier was hanged.

Another case in which a strychnine poisoner almost escaped

occurred in April 1929, in Tittletown, California. First World War veteran Carroll Rablen and his pretty wife Eva had attended a dance at the local school-house. Because of a war injury, Carroll Rablen was deaf, and so could not hear the music, but he sat outside in his car while his wife, who was a keen dancer, went inside.

About midnight, Eva pushed through the crowd outside the school-house with a cup of coffee and some sandwiches for her husband, handed them to him, and went back to the festivities; Carroll took a large gulp of the coffee and seconds later began to writhe and let out choked cries of agony. Several people, among them his father, ran to his aid while someone went for a doctor. But it was too late; Carroll managed to tell his father that the coffee tasted bitter, and then collapsed and died.

Eva appeared to be distraught with grief, and neighbours recalled to the police that the injured ex-soldier had talked of suicide some time previously, but although the contents of his stomach were analysed by a chemist in a nearby town, no trace of poison was found. The police discovered, however, that insurance on Rablen's life, made out to Eva, totalled $3000, and they began systematically to search the area around the school-house. They were successful – under a wood-pile was a broken bottle with the label 'Strychnine' and the name of a local chemist on it. The pharmacist traced the poison sale in his register; it had been made three days before Rablen's death to a woman giving her name as Mrs Joe Williams, who said she wanted it to kill gophers. Although the chemist identified Mrs Rablen with 'Mrs Williams' and Eva was arrested, the police case looked weak, because of the failure of analysis to show strychnine in Rablen's stomach. Then Dr Edward Heinrich, an eminent medico-legal examiner, was called in to help. He found minute traces of the poison in Rablen's stomach, but more importantly he discovered traces of strychnine crystals in the coffee cup. Pondering the circumstances of the case, he realized that Eva must have had an extremely steady hand to push through the jostling crowd carrying the coffee without spilling any. Perhaps she had splashed a bystander? The police appealed for anyone who remembered being jostled by Eva that night, and a woman came forward. Her stained dress contained traces of strychnine, and confronted with the evidence, Eva Rablen confessed and was sentenced to life imprisonment.

With the gradual control of the 'old fashioned' poisons such as arsenic, cyanide, and strychnine, criminological toxicologists felt for a while that they had earned a respite; unfortunately this was not so. The widespread use of barbiturates after the Second World War and their relative availability on prescription caused a rise in suicides, which alarmed the medical profession; in 1954 there were 12 times the number of known barbiturate suicides than there had been in 1938. A year after these figures were produced a particularly tragic case provided the world with the first known homicide by barbiturate.

Early in the morning of 22 July 1955, a 26-year-old male nurse named John Armstrong of Gosport, near Portsmouth, who worked in a local naval hospital, called his medical practitioner Dr Bernard Johnson to say that his five-month-old son Terence was very ill. Dr Johnson knew Armstrong and his wife Janet, aged 19, well. They had two other children besides Terence, and like most young couples the strain of three children often caused them to be in minor debt. Coupled to the strain of debt they had suffered tragedy; their first child Stephen had died in March 1954, and their two-year-old daughter Pamela had suffered a sudden illness in May the same year, but had recovered in hospital.

When Dr Johnson arrived at the house he found that the baby had died and, although he did not suspect foul play, he could not identify the cause of death, and accordingly notified the Gosport coroner. The body, the baby's bottle, and a pillow he had vomited onto the previous evening were taken to the mortuary to be examined by pathologist Dr Harold Miller.

Examining the larynx, Dr Miller found a shrivelled red shell which reminded him of the skin of a daphne berry – a highly poisonous fruit. In the child's stomach were further shells. He placed the shell from the daphne berry in a bottle of formaldehyde, and the rest of the stomach contents in another bottle, and stored the two containers in a refrigerator.

By now he was convinced that berry poisoning had caused

death, and asked the coroner's office to ask if the child had had access to the berries. The coroner's officer called on the Armstrongs and to his shocked surprise found them watching television as if nothing had happened. Neverthless he found a fruiting daphne tree in the garden, and Armstrong remembered that the child's pram had stood under it. The officer reported back to Dr Miller.

Dr Miller was convinced that his first idea had been correct, until he opened the refrigerator to find that the shell in the formaldehyde had disappeared and the shells in the other bottle had also vanished, dyeing the stomach contents red. Dr Miller now sent both bottles, along with the pillow and feeding bottle, to a chemical laboratory, which reported back that there was no sign of any poison, and no trace of the daphne berry skin; the only unusual features were a small quantity of cornstarch and a red dye, eosin.

Dr Miller pondered the problem, and realized that such a combination could be found in red medical capsules, for instance those used to contain the barbiturate seconal. He dissolved seconal capsules in gastric juices and found that they reduced themselves to cornstarch and eosin. He knew that there was no precedent for murder by barbiturates, but also that a few grains of seconal would be enough to kill an infant. When he reported the facts to the police, Superintendent L. C. Nicholls, Director of Scotland Yard's Forensic Laboratory, was called in. After tests lasting five days he discovered that the vomit traces on the pillow contained 1/50th of a grain of seconal, while he also found one third of a grain in the stomach.

Meanwhile, Gosport police, alerted by Superintendent Nicholls's preliminary report, went to the naval hospital where Armstrong worked and asked if any seconal had gone missing; they discovered a nurse who worked on the same floor as Armstrong and who remembered the mysterious disappearance of fifty 1½ grain seconal capsules from a cupboard to which Armstrong had access.

With this admittedly circumstantial evidence to hand, the police opened enquiries into the boy Stephen's death the previous year; his death had been certified by an 82-year-old doctor who had not known the family, but the symptoms had been the same suffered by Terence – blue tinged face, drowsiness, breathing difficulty and death. Furthermore two-year-old Pamela's sudden illness had taken the same course.

Finally, with Superintendent Nicholls's report that he had found a total of 1/20th of a grain of seconal in the dead baby – from which he deduced that at least three to five capsules had been administered – an exhumation order was granted for the body of Stephen. Unfortunately, decomposition had destroyed all traces of any relevant chemical in the remains.

Nicholls had by now begun experimenting on the time taken for the seconal capsule of the type administered to baby Terence to burst in the stomach. He found that the methyl cellulose which, dyed with eosin, made up the capsule, absorbed stomach fluids and caused cornstarch in the interior to swell; this in turn caused the capsule to burst open and discharge the contents into the stomach. The whole process took up to ninety minutes, and while he was not convinced that the Armstrongs were guilty, he had to prove that they were in possession of seconal on the day of the murder.

It was a year later before he had his evidence. In July 1956 Janet Armstrong applied for a separation order against her husband, on the grounds that he had beaten her up repeatedly; the order was refused and she spitefully went to the Gosport police and told them that her husband had had seconal capsules in his possession on the day of the murder. In December the same year, faced with this elaborate and at that time unique evidence, a judge acquitted Janet but found John Armstrong guilty of murdering his child.

A few months after the conclusion of the Armstrong case, in May 1957, another 'first' for toxicologists occurred, which was to rival the Armstrong case in complexity. At around midnight on 3 May, a thirty-eight-year-old man named Kenneth Barlow – like Armstrong a male nurse – asked a neighbour to call a doctor to his home in Thornbury Crescent, Bradford. His wife Elizabeth had died in the bath, he said. When the doctor arrived Barlow told him that his wife had been sick all evening and had vomited in bed at about 9.30. She had decided to have a bath and he had gone to bed and dosed off to sleep, after changing the sheets.

When he awoke at 11 pm he found that his wife was not beside him and hurried to the bathroom. There he had found his wife apparently drowned, and despite frantic attempts to pull her out and revive her with artificial respiration, had been unable to do so. The doctor found the body lying in the empty bath – Barlow had pulled the plug – on her right side. She had apparently vomited, and though there were no signs of violence on the body the eyes were dilated. The doctor called the police. Barlow repeated his story, and the police called in forensic experts. They too noted the dilated pupils, a possible sign of poisoning. Moreover the police noticed the fact that although Barlow claimed to have made 'frantic efforts' to save his wife, his pyjamas were dry and there was no sign of splashing on the bathroom floor; further, a sharp-eyed detective spotted that there was water in the crooks of Mrs Barlow's elbows, which threw doubts on the theory that artificial respiration had been administered.

Two hypodermic syringes were found in the kitchen, which Barlow explained by saying that he had been treating himself for a carbuncle with penicillin. He was after all a nurse at Bradford Royal Infirmary. He denied giving his wife any injections.

The syringes and the body were removed for post-mortem, which only left the medical examiners baffled. Traces of penicillin in the needles seemed to bear out Barlow's story, but they could find no trace of poison or drugs in the body, and despite being two months pregnant Mrs Barlow had been disease free and completely healthy. However, with the aid of a hand lens, they went over every inch of the dead woman's skin, looking for marks of injection; Mrs Barlow was liberally freckled which made the task a difficult one, but finally two tell-tale puncture marks were found on the right buttock and another two, more recent, in the fold of skin under the left buttock. An incision made into the latter showed up characteristic inflammation, suggesting that an injection had indeed been made only a short time before death. But what had been injected? A conference of doctors, chemists and forensic experts was called to consider the baffling facts. Barlow the nurse had confidently and efficiently described his wife's symptoms to them immediately prior to death – vomiting, sweating, and weakness. There was the dilation of the eyes, too, to be considered. All evidence described hypoglycaemia – a deficiency of blood sugar and a characteristic of 'insulin shock'.

But here the pathologists came up against a stone wall; Mrs Barlow was not diabetic, and an examination of heart blood showed an above average level of sugar – the opposite of what could be expected to happen had she been given insulin. To make things more difficult, there were no prescribed tests for detecting insulin in the body tissues. The team of forensic experts went back to grass roots and began searching every medical textbook and paper on the effects of insulin known. Finally they came up with a solution which at least seemed to solve the high level of sugar in the heart. The phenomenon, it appeared, had been noticed in several cases of violent death, and biochemical research had shown that this was due to the liver assisting survival by discharging a heavy dose of sugar into the bloodstream moments before death; this reached the heart before circulation stopped, and consequently the heart blood was high in blood sugar.

In the case of Mrs Barlow, therefore, she could have been given insulin. Now they began experiments with mice in an attempt to isolate the substance in her blood. A number of mice were injected with insulin in a controlled experiment; they trembled, made weak noises, went into coma and died. Then extracts of the tissue surrounding the injection marks on the woman's body were injected into similar mice – exactly the same reaction was observed. Specifically, mice injected with matter from the left, recently marked buttock, died quicker than those given tissue from the right. Judging by this and other facts, doctors and chemists estimated that the quantity of the drug remaining in the body was 84 units, but the actual dosage must have been much higher.

One obstacle remained: up until then the common belief among doctors – and nurses, who, like Barlow, injected patients with insulin – was that the substance disappeared very quickly from the body. But new research came to the aid of the examiners. It was known that acidic conditions preserved insulin, and it now appeared that formation of lactic acid in Mrs Barlow's muscles after death had prevented its breakdown. Chemical changes in the muscles after death were known to produce lactic acid, but never before had it been necessary to relate this to the injection of insulin.

Meanwhile, Bradford police had been investigating Mr Barlow's background. They discovered that he had been married previously, and that his first wife had died in 1956 aged 33. The cause of death had never been satisfactorily explained, and he had married Elizabeth shortly afterwards. More damning, he had often injected insulin at the Infirmary, and had once joked to a patient: 'If anybody ever gets a real dose of this, he's on his way to the next world.'

On 29 July 1957, Barlow was arrested and charged with murdering his wife by giving her an overdose of insulin. For a while he persisted in denying that he had injected her at any time, and then 'confessed' to having given her a dose of ergonovine to induce an abortion. In fact the forensic experts had made a thorough check for abortifacient drugs at the post-mortem; none had been found.

At Barlow's trial the only medical defence put up was that Mrs Barlow had, in her weakness, slid under the bath water and in a moment of fear her body had reacted by injecting a massive dose of insulin into the bloodstream, causing coma and death. This theory was briskly dealt with by one of the expert biochemists. He reckoned that to account for the 84 units of insulin in Mrs Barlow's body her pancreas would have had to secrete an incredible – and quite impossible – 15,000 units.

For their work, the team of scientific experts received high commendation from the judge and the happy knowledge that they had added another dimension to modern forensic science. For his part, Kenneth Barlow received life imprisonment.

The Armstrong and Barlow cases illustrate the recurring nightmare of most toxicologists today: that a case of poisoning will go unrecognized as such, leading its perpetrator to further crime as he gathers confidence. Though there are now tight restrictions on inorganic and synthetic poisons, the organic varieties – vegetable poisons such as belladonna and various fungi – are almost impossible to control, for they grow wild in many areas of Europe and the United States. Also difficult are those drugs, rarely if ever used in homicide, which nevertheless are deadly when not used for their specific purpose, in industry, for instance.

Add to these dangers the possibility of a psychopathic killer with access to and a knowledge of poisons, and the forces of law are in grave straits. The odds against such a combination of factors seem steep, but they did occur in Britain during the summer of 1971.

The John Hadland Laboratories at Bovingdon in Hertfordshire, sited in green countryside some miles north of London and manufacturing photographic equipment, seemed to be one of the happiest of all possible working environments. The firm's managing director, Godfrey Foster, encouraged close relationships between shop-floor employees and management and any problems which arose were usually thrashed out in an atmosphere of communal respect.

One of the best respected of all Hadland employees was 60-year-old Bob Egle, head storeman at the firm. Mr Egle was fit and active, and looked forward to his forthcoming retirement. Then in July 1971, he began to suffer spasms of pain in his chest and back. Food and drink tended to make him vomit, and his sense of balance was impaired. His doctor diagnosed some disorder of the nervous system, and treated him for peripheral neuritis, but he continued to deteriorate and was eventually lodged in the intensive care unit of the St Alban's City Hospital. There, on 19 July, he died.

Mr Foster naturally decided to attend the funeral of his long-serving employee, and chose 23-year-old Graham Young, the newest member of his staff and one of Mr Egle's assistants, to accompany him as a representative of Hadland's rank and file. On the way, they talked of Mr Egle's illness. Later, Mr Foster recalled his surprise at Graham's medical knowledge. He had mentioned that the death certificate noted peripheral neuritis as a contributing factor. Young commented:

That is just a general term meaning that the illness affected the whole nervous system. He probably suffered from the Guillain-Barre Syndrome, and the terminal cause of death was almost certainly broncho-pneumonia.

In fact Young knew the details of Egle's death because he had been studying them for some years. Since childhood he had been an avid reader of toxicological textbooks, and in 1962 had been committed to Broadmoor, the institution for the criminally insane, after admitting to killing his step-mother with poison and attempting to poison his father, his sister, and a school friend.

In February 1971 he had been released after the authorities decided that there was little chance of his reverting to his 'hobby' of poisoning, and after a spell in a rehabilitation centre he had applied for his job at Hadland's. He had told the friendly Godfrey Foster that he had suffered a 'nervous breakdown' after leaving school; Mr Foster was impressed by him, and had taken him onto the workforce.

By pure chance an outbreak of gastro-enteritis had afflicted the school children of the Bovingdon area at the time Young had joined Hadland's; the epidemic was so bad that the villagers termed it the 'Bovingdon bug'. It appears to have rekindled the urge to poison in Graham Young's mind, and at Hadland's he had the means to hand – a relatively rare compound of thallium, used in the manufacture of camera lenses. In minute quantities thallium salts had been used by the medical profession in the treatment of ringworm and as a depilatory, but even this use was discontinued in the 1940s because of the drastic results of even a small accidental dose.

Young had used a thallium compound to kill Bob Egle, lacing his tea with it, and in October, just over three months after Egle's death, he began systematically to poison his replacement, a 56-year-old man named Fred Biggs. In the last week in October, Biggs was seized with what appeared to be a dose of the 'Bovingdon bug' for two days running. He was able to report for overtime on Saturday 30 October, however, and when he arrived at the stores shed he was met by Graham Young, who had made him a friendly cup of tea.

Young recorded his acts in a meticulously kept diary. That night he wrote: 'I have administered a fatal dose of the special compound to F [Fred] and anticipate a report of his progress on Monday, 1st November, I gave him three separate doses.'

Like Egle, Fred Biggs mystified the local doctors, and was eventually moved to the National Hospital for Nervous Diseases, in London, where he died on 19 November. The fighting spirit which kept him alive for so long irritated Young.

He is surviving too long for my peace of mind. It is better that he should die. It will be a merciful release for him, as if he should survive he will be permanently impaired.

After the death of Fred Biggs, Young singled out two more victims, Jethro Batt and David Tilson. Over a period of time Batt was fed about four grains of the poison – 12 being calculated as the lethal dose – and Tilson received between five and six grains. Both of them suffered chest pains and numbness in the legs, but to Young's alarm they also developed 'side symptoms' – their hair began to fall out. According to his diary he was concerned that doctors would suspect thallium poisoning – thallium having a depilatory effect – and trace it back to him.

'I must watch this situation very carefully,' he wrote. 'If it looks like I will be detected then I shall have to destroy myself.'

Though both Batt and Tilson survived, Godfrey Foster was

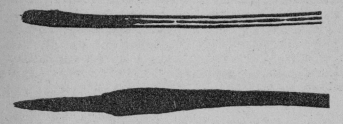

*Compared with a normal hair (top) a hair from one of Graham Young's victims shows characteristic distortion indicating thallium poisoning (Metropolitan Police).*

becoming alarmed and called in a team of toxicologists, headed by Dr Andrew Anderson. It was not a forensic enquiry; Foster was convinced that through some leakage of the chemicals used in his plant, his staff were being accidentally poisoned. He told Dr Anderson of the friendly staff relationships at Hadland's and suggested he call a meeting with the employees. When the doctor did so, offering to answer questions, his first interrogator was Graham Young, who asked him if he did not think that the symptoms of Egle, Biggs, Batt and Tilson were consistent with thallium poisoning?

Dr Anderson was intrigued. Thallium, though mentioned in standard textbooks, is a rare drug where homicide is concerned. He studied its reported effects, and found that they did coincide with the symptoms of the 'Bovingdon bug' victims. He also made enquiries about the young man who seemed to know so much about poisons, and eventually asked Scotland Yard to check their records for any trace of him.

Of course, Young's record as a former Broadmoor inmate was on file, and he was immediately arrested. At first, even confronted with his diary, he denied all knowledge of the crimes, claiming that the diary was merely notes for a novel. Then the police found a dose of thallium in the lining of his coat. He told them that it was his 'exit dose' and that he had intended to kill himself with it if discovered; he also admitted killing Egle and Biggs, and said that he could have killed four others – 'but I let them live'.

In June 1972, Young was sentenced to life imprisonment at St. Albans. In mitigation, his defence counsel said that his mind had been affected by the death of his mother three months after he was born. The truth is that no one knows precisely what activates people like Graham Young. All forensic scientists can do is study the effects of their work – and hope for a swift solution.

# Chapter Twelve

# A face from the past

E'en from the tomb the voice of nature cries
E'en in our ashes live their wonted fires.

Thomas Gray, *Elegy written in a country churchyard*

In the late 1920s, the Swedish authorities approached Sir Bernard Spilsbury with a curious problem. They had discovered the embalmed body of James Hepburn, Earl of Bothwell, the third husband of Mary Queen of Scots. The body had lain in the vaults of Malmö castle for almost four hundred years, ever since the hapless nobleman had been imprisoned there for piracy, and the Swedes wanted to know just how he had died.

Reluctantly and politely, Sir Bernard told them that he could not help. As fastidious as ever on matters touching his career and reputation, he explained that he could not be certain of pin-pointing the exact cause of death after the passage of such a time, and if he could not guarantee precision he preferred not to give any opinion at all.

He had been ill at the time, and perhaps this, and the constant pressure of his regular work, influenced his decision. Whatever the cause, the great pathologist was almost certainly being over cautious, and doing himself less than justice. For, in several cases, forensic surgeons had already been called in to examine the remains of long dead people, to identify them or establish the cause of death, and in the years to come forensic science was to play a dramatic role in assisting archaeologists and historians in this way.

Perhaps the most spectacular of such cases occurred during the 1960s, when the process of neutron activation analysis was used in an attempt to show whether or not Napoleon Bonaparte had died of natural causes. The experiment was not absolutely conclusive, but it set historians – French ones in particular – thinking again about the death of the great Emperor-warrior.

Just before his death in exile on the British colony of St Helena in 1821. Napoleon had written in his will: 'I am dying before my time, murdered by the English oligarchy and its hired assassin' – apparently a reference to the island's governor, General Sir Hudson Lowe. When the Emperor died, an Italian surgeon performed an autopsy on his body and pronounced the cause of death to be stomach cancer. The body was buried on the island and lay there undisturbed for almost twenty years until, in 1840, it was shipped back to France for reinterment in the great tomb-monument of Les Invalides in Paris.

The French had always been uneasy about the circumstances of Napoleon's last days; there was the accusation in the will, and there were the persistent stories, little more than legend, that he had in fact been poisoned by his companion and attendant Count Montholon, who had received two million francs under the terms of the Emperor's will.

When neutron activation analysis became available, forensic experts subjected hair clipped from Napoleon's head as a memento, along with a few hairs which had been embedded in his death mask, to the test. The results showed that the hair contained 13 times the amount of arsenic normally contained in human hair, and that he had taken arsenic at least 40 times in the months immediately preceding his death.

Despite the evidence of the tests, opponents of the murder theory pointed out that several factors might well have added to the arsenical content of the Emperor's remains. The body could have absorbed the chemical from the soil at St Helena during its 19-year burial there; he could have taken small quantities of arsenic as a stimulant; and he could have been treated with medicines in which arsenic was an ingredient, for the substance was widely used in medications until the end of the nineteenth century.

Counter to these theories ran the fact that absorption of the chemical in such quantity was unlikely to have occurred from the sources suggested and also that the body, when disinterred in 1840 for removal to Paris, was almost perfectly preserved, a typical feature of corpses which have been poisoned with arsenic. Apart from slight decay at the tip of the nose and the rims of the ears it remained unchanged; the condition was so good that a second death mask could be taken from it.

It was this second mask which was brought into the argument

after the neutron activation findings were announced, with results which shook all France. A Napoleonic authority, Georges Restif de la Bretonne, claimed that the body in Les Invalides was not Napoleon at all but was his butler, one Cipriani, who had committed suicide on St Helena three years before the Emperor's death. The British, claimed Restif de la Bretonne, had never had any intention of giving up Napoleon's corpse; instead they had secretly removed it for burial in the undercoft of Westminster Abbey in 1828, substituting the corpse of the dead butler in the St Helena grave.

Preposterous as the theory sounded, the two death masks had to be explained away. The one taken at the time of Napoleon's death is that of a slightly wrinkled old man with plump jowls; the other, made from the body dug up for reinterment in Paris, is of a hollow-cheeked, thin-faced individual who bears a striking resemblance to portraits of Cipriani. So far the French authorities have refused applications for the re-opening of the tomb in Les Invalides. Until such time as they do so, giving medical experts the opportunity to probe deeper into the mystery, French patriots will be left with the nagging question: does the splendid marble tomb in Paris contain the body of a mere servant?

A much more satisfactory conclusion was put, in 1968, to the hundred-year-old mystery surrounding the death of the American polar explorer Captain Charles Francis Hall. Again the case involved arsenic, and again neutron activation analysis was brought into play.

Born in 1820, the son of a New Hampshire blacksmith, Charles Hall was largely self-taught. Once he had mastered reading, however, he devoured books voraciously, particularly accounts of polar exploration, which fascinated him. He became obsessed with the mystery of the disappearance of Sir John Franklin and members of his expedition, who had vanished with their ship, HMS *Erebus*, some years earlier in 1847. Hall determined to visit the Arctic, teach himself Eskimo, and try to discover the fate of the British party. During two expeditions, lasting a total of seven years, he succeeded remarkably well, for although he did not find Franklin's body itself, he came across a number of other skeletons, among them that of Lieutenant Le Vesconte, second in command of the *Erebus*, which was later returned to Greenwich, London, for burial. Hall also found traces of a house built by Martin Frobisher, the Elizabethan explorer, and his account of this discovery, which he wrote for the American newspapers, made him into a popular hero. He was, therefore, a natural choice as leader when Congress authorized President Ulysses S. Grant to send an American expedition in search of the North Pole. On 3 July 1871, Hall commanded the 387-ton steam tug *Polaris* as it sailed out of New London, Connecticut, on the first leg of the voyage.

To his crew, Captain Hall was a hero whom they worshipped. Unfortunately the big, bearded commander did not get on quite so well with his officers. His second-in-command, Captain Sidney Buddington, had been pressed into the expedition against his will, and did not take kindly to Hall dressing him down when he was caught stealing whisky from the supply cupboard. But Hall's main trouble came from the leader of the scientific party, Dr Emil Bessels, a twenty-four-year-old German who also served as ship's physician. An intellectual snob, he looked down on the rest of the party, particularly on Captain Hall. On several occasions, the captain – who, during his Frobisher expedition, had shot and killed a sailor who disobeyed him – came down on Dr Bessels with a heavy hand. Everyone on board the *Polaris* knew of the dislike which existed between the two men.

By the beginning of September, the *Polaris* had reached the northern coast of Greenland, and Captain Hall anchored in an inlet which he named Thank God Harbour, and snugged the vessel down for winter, while he himself, accompanied by faithful Eskimos, made several forays by dog sleigh to map out a route for the coming spring.

On the afternoon of 24 October, Captain Hall returned from a scouting trip and called for hot coffee. At a subsequent inquiry, there was a clash of testimony as to the origin of the coffee he received; one witness said that it came from the simmering galley pot, while another held that it had been specially brewed for the captain. In any case, he drank only half a cup and then began to vomit, doubled over with pain. Dr Bessels came and asked him about his symptoms. Hall managed to gasp: 'Pain in the stomach, burning, and my legs feel weak.'

Bessels examined him, and then confided in his fellow officers that Captain Hall was suffering from an attack of apoplexy, from which it was unlikely that he would recover. That evening Hall's friend and assistant navigator, Captain George Tyson, wrote in his diary: 'Captain Hall is sick; it is strange, and he looked so well . . . this sickness came on immediately after drinking a cup of coffee.'

The following day, the stricken captain seemed to rally a little, but later suffered further attacks, despite, as Tyson noted, Dr Bessels giving him 'frequent medication'. By 3 November the captain had gone into a definite decline; he 'talked wildly' to Tyson about being poisoned, and called 'for first one and then the other, as if he did not know who to trust'.

In his more lucid periods, Captain Hall was seen making notes in his private journals – which disappeared in mysterious circumstances some time later, allegedly thrown overboard to lighten ship. On one such occasion he turned to Captain Buddington and asked: 'Tell me Sidney, how do you spell murder?'

Bessels, too, approached Buddington with a problem: Hall would no longer take the medication he prescribed. Buddington suggested that the doctor should make up a larger dose, so that he, Buddington, could take the first spoonful and so reassure the Captain. Bessels hastily refused. At the inquiry it was also revealed that Bessels took to giving Hall injections of a liquid which he distilled from 'little white crystals'.

Late in the evening of 7 November, Hall seemed to give up all efforts of will. As several officers stood around his bunk, he opened his eyes and looked at Bessels. 'Doctor,' he said calmly, 'I am very much obliged to you for your kindness.' He then lapsed into a coma and died some hours later.

Almost all the ship's company were devastated by the news; but not quite all. Captain Buddington told a seaman, after Hall's burial: 'That's a stone off my heart.' Both Bessels and his assistant Meyer, who had also fallen foul of Hall, became what must have seemed indecently lighthearted.

At eleven o'clock on the morning of 10 November 1871, Hall was wrapped in the American flag, placed in a coffin made by the ship's carpenter, and buried in a shallow grave on the frozen shores of Thank God Harbour.

For the next ten months the *Polaris*, now with Captain Buddington in command, lay locked in ice floes. In the following August, after a few tentative expeditions by dog sleigh had been attempted, Buddington broke the ship free of the ice and began the long voyage southwards. For two months, hampered by floating icebergs, the ship drifted, and then in October disaster struck. The *Polaris* was lying in Smith Sound when she was nipped between two large bergs. The crew tossed supplies and other equipment overboard onto an ice floe and abandoned what they thought was the sinking ship. But with her load lightened, she broke away and quickly drifted out of sight.

The saga of how the party managed, by trekking from one ice patch to another, to make for safety is a noble chapter in the history of American exploration. Under the guidance of Captain Tyson the navigator, and fed on seal meat by the Eskimos, the group made its way to the coast of Labrador, where it was rescued by an American whaling ship on 30 April 1873.

That summer a four-man panel sat for the inquiry into the fate of Captain Hall in Washington, under the guidance of the Secretary for the United States Navy, George Robeson. After hearing the evidence of all the witnesses, they ruled that Captain Hall had died from apoplexy, and that his death was 'without fault on the part of anyone'.

But for almost a hundred years, doubts remained as to the true circumstances of Hall's sudden decease. Finally, in August 1968, Professor Chauncey C. Loomis of Dartmouth College, New Hampshire, Hall's home state, and pathologist F. K. Paddock of Pittsfield, Massachusetts, flew from Resolute Bay in Canada's North West Territories to find the grave and examine the body. The site had been marked by a tablet of oak and brass; after a few minutes digging, the Loomis party uncovered the coffin in its shallow grave, and prised off the lid. The whole thing, body and coffin alike, was frozen into the permafrost, and Dr Paddock had to perform his autopsy half squatting astride the hole in what must be one of the most uncomfortable post-mortems on record.

The body, clad in a Captain's uniform and draped in the slightly faded flag, was remarkably well preserved. Apart from empty eye sockets and a shrivelled nose tip, the face was intact, and the rust-red beard and hair had lost none of its colouring. Although most of the internal organs had shrivelled, the trunk and limbs of the body had undergone the adipocere change from long lying in the moist atmosphere.

Dr Paddock carefully removed a section of skull, along with amorphous tissue from what remained of the brain and heart area; he also recovered samples from the hair and beard, a fingernail and a fingertip, and soil samples from the grave area. This material was sent first to the Public Safety Laboratory, Boston, and then to the Centre of Forensic Sciences, Toronto. The hair was subjected to neutron activation in the nuclear reactor at MacMaster University, Hamilton.

Douglas M. Lucas, Director of the Toronto laboratory, was able to show that a high concentration of arsenic was present in the root of the fingernail, as compared with the amount at the tip. Similar results were obtained from the hair samples. He explained:

Assuming average growth rates of fingernails and hair, these results show that elevated amounts of arsenic had been deposited in the nails and hair during the last two to five weeks of Hall's life, with the highest amounts being incorporated into the nails and hair within one week of his death.

Arsenic content in the soil samples from the burial site was high, 'but', explained Lucas:

Hair and nail samples were washed before irradiation. Had arsenic come from the soil, it would have been distributed uniformly. In neither fingernail nor hair was this the case . . . In any case of suspected homicidal poisoning, the symptoms attending death are of prime importance. The symptoms Hall was alleged to have are characteristic of arsenic poisoning . . . On the strength of our analysis alone I would not be as certain as I am – if there had not been the symptoms. When you look at the two I think you have to reach the conclusion that arsenic poisoning is a fair diagnosis.

As a corollary to Lucas's findings, and in view of the testimony given at the inquiry, it seems not over assumptive to name Hall's murderer: Dr Emil Bessels, the jealous young snob who appeared to attend the captain so carefully, and then rejoiced in his death.

Not all cases in which modern forensic techniques are used to delve into the past are concerned with causes of death. In one striking instance, the late Professor Mikhail Gerasimov, whose facial reconstruction techniques, enhancing the prestige of Russian forensic technology, have already been described, was able to show probable motive for the brutal actions of one of the most famous despots of all time.

On 23 April 1953, Gerasimov was a member of a special commission from the Soviet Ministry of Culture which, under the direction of Professor A. N. Smirnov, opened the sarcophagus of Tsar Ivan IV in the Archangel Cathedral which forms part of the Kremlin.

Ivan Grozni, 'The Terrible', acceded to the principality of Moscow in 1533, when he was three years old, and showed sadistic streaks in his character even at this tender age. By the time he was crowned first Tsar of All the Russians in 1547, his murderous rages, drunken acts of cruelty, and indiscriminate sexual passions had earned him his soubriquet. Yet as a ruler his character was full of contradictions; he brought about much needed land and church reforms, consolidated Russia's borders to the East, and opened up diplomatic relationships with England. After the desertion of his confidant Prince Kurbsky in 1564 to the King of Poland, Ivan instigated a reign of terror which lasted until his death in 1584; this culminated, three years before he died, with the murder of his heir by his own hand. Such was the man whose corpse Gerasimov and Smirnov set out to seek.

Like all tombs in the Archangel Cathedral, that of Ivan was sheathed with bronze; below this was a layer of plaster, which covered the brickwork of the tomb itself. The investigators penetrated the brick, and underneath discovered the white stone sarcophagus of the Tsar.

The body lay with its arms crossed over its breast, and was clad in the dusty remains of a monk's habit, on which were embroidered the texts of prayers. A crucifixion scene, worked in coloured silk, adorned a cloth over the torso, but as if to set off this evidence of belated piety, a drinking goblet of dark blue glass enamelled in yellow stood to the left of the head.

Adhering to the brittle skull bones were a few traces of hair from the eyebrows and beard. The Tsar had been a fairly tall man of around six feet in height; according to contemporary reports he had been very strong in his youth, but towards the end of his life put on weight until he eventually tipped the scales at 210 pounds.

Carefully stripped of its robes, the skeleton in the tomb told a clear tale of suffering to the scientists. Quite early in his life, Ivan's cartilages and ligaments had begun to ossify, or harden, and the joints of the long bones all showed traces of inflammation leading to the conclusion that he had suffered from polyarthritis. Almost the whole skeleton showed signs of the torsion which accompanies this disease.

Chemical analysis revealed the presence of arsenic and mercury in the body; the arsenic content was judged to be normal, but the mercury count was very high. The scientists concluded that a quicksilver-based ointment had been used regularly in an attempt to alleviate the pain in his limbs.

To add to the misery of his bone disease Tsar Ivan had undergone an extremely painful and very rare experience during his fifties – at the peak of his 'reign of terror'. Judging by the state of his teeth, his adult, or secondary incisors, canines and premolars had only come through the gums at this late time, and the process must have been an agonising one.

All this did not excuse the behaviour of Ivan the Terrible, but it did go a long way towards explaining it. As a youth he had a tendency to be cruel, and the perpetual pain of his adult life, coupled with his heavy drinking in an effort to alleviate it, could only have led to a savage warping of his already embittered character.

It now fell to Professor Gerasimov to reconstruct the features of the dead tyrant. 'In order to free myself from the numerous representations of the Tsar,' he wrote, 'I chose deliberately a more complicated technique than usual in my reconstruction.'

After making a plaster cast of the delicate skull and torso bones, he reconstructed the deep lying muscles of the neck and head; the whole process was filmed and photographed.

The most revealing portrait was that of the face without any hair. It seemed to hide nothing – the form of the low forehead, the peculiarities of the supraorbital area, the size and outline of the symmetrical orbits which conditioned the external specific appearance of the eyes. The mouth with its drooping corners and expression of disgust was determined by the shape of the dentition. The face was hard, commanding, undoubtedly clever but cruel and unpleasing, with pendulous nose and clumsy chin.

The portrait reconstructed from the skull, he concluded, agreed exactly with the descriptions his contemporaries gave of the appearance of Tsar Ivan IV.

In perhaps the most brilliant case of forensic archaeology on record, the object was to achieve something quite as dramatic: to prove the identity of the little pile of damaged bones believed to be those of Edward of England, Saxon King and Martyr.

During the reign of King Edgar, between the years AD 959 and 975 in England, the established church was split into two factions. On the one hand were the monks of the great abbeys and religious houses, dedicated to improving the quality of life; on the other were the 'secular' clergy, bishops and priests who made fortunes from the administration of their parishes and spent the money in high living. Many of the nobles supported the latter factions for their own ends, although at least two – the northern King Oswald and Bishop Dunstan, who were both destined to become saints – fought for the reformation and unification of the Church.

King Edgar himself, despite his own tendency towards the profligate, supported the monks and built 40 great monasteries during his lifetime; when he died, his fifteen-year-old son Edward took up the cause, backed by Oswald and Dunstan. But Edward was to reign for only four years. In his eighteenth summer, while on a visit to his younger brother Aethelred – later to be dubbed 'the Unready' – at what is now Corfe Castle, Dorset, Edward was ambushed and murdered.

A monk in Edward's entourage at the time of the attack later wrote an account of the slaying in his *Life of St Oswald* in about AD 1000.

Soldiers were therefore holding him, one drew him (the King) to the right toward himself as though to give him a kiss (of welcome) another seized his left hand violently and wounded him, but he cried as loud as he could 'What are you doing, breaking my right arm?' and he fell from his horse and died.

The report, written, of course, in Latin, gives a detailed picture of the assassination. Two soldiers approached the King on horseback, one to the left, the other to the right. The latter grasped Edward's left shoulder with his own right arm and drew the King towards him for the kiss of peace; at the same time he got a grip on the King's right forearm – the sword arm – with his left hand.

As soon as the King was pinioned like this, and momentarily helpless, the soldier on his left twisted his left arm and stabbed him with a knife. The King's horse reared up in panic and forced its royal rider back onto the high cantle of the saddle, and with the two attackers still holding him the young King's thigh was pressed hard across the cantle.

Then the horse bolted, throwing Edward from the saddle and dragging him along the ground by his left foot, which was caught in the stirrup; by the time his faithful followers caught and calmed his mount, the King was dead. Within a few days his treacherous younger brother Aethelred had mounted the throne to begin his own unfortunate reign.

Like those of his companions Oswald and Dunstan, Edward's violent end was considered to be martyrdom, and he was canonized as 'Saint Edward the Martyr'; his shrine at Shaftesbury Abbey became a popular place of pilgrimage and was a favourite resort of worshippers until the dissolution of the monastic system by Henry VIII in the sixteenth century.

At that time the richly-worked tomb was smashed, and the body of the dead King, like that of many another early English saint, appeared to be lost forever. Then, on 2 January 1931, a pious archaeologist named J. Wilson Claridge discovered a lead casket containing bones on the site of the Shaftesbury Abbey church.

The casket was 21 inches long, 11 inches wide, and 9 inches deep; the bones had been neatly arranged, with the small ones at the bottom, the long ones at one side, and part of a skull on top. Claridge was convinced that these were the mortal remains of St Edward. Accordingly, he brought in Dr Thomas E. A. Stowell, FRCS, a distinguished forensic pathologist.

Stowell's first inspection of the remains was encouraging. They were, he said, the bones of a person who had sustained a remarkable number of 'greenstick' fractures – breakages which only occur in the pliable bones of the young. The British Museum Department of Anthropology reinforced the remains with synthetic resin, and then handed them over for examination.

Stowell began by measuring the remaining long bones of the arms and legs. Making allowances for scalp and heel pad thickness, and estimating various characteristics from the other bones, he was able to say that the dead person had been between five feet six and five feet eight inches in height.

Then he set out to discover the sex. There are several methods of 'sexing' a skeleton. The shape of the pelvis is usually the most indicative, but the sacrum – the wedge-shaped bone at the bottom of the spine – and the femur, or thigh bone, are also important. The skull can provide data, and there are 'mathematical' methods of establishing sex by measuring the heads or thick ends of the humerus, upper arm bone, or femur. Stowell found that the body had been that of a male. Now he needed to know its race. The skull, he decided – from the fragments remaining – was 'dolichocephalic', or long-headed. The Saxons were long-headed, whereas the Britons and Celts were 'round-headed'. So it was reasonable to suppose that the remains were Saxon.

The vertebrae were revealing too. In the neck there are normally seven of these bones, but the casket contained only the first, second, and seventh; the missing third, fourth, fifth and sixth appeared to have disintegrated, and by following up further clues Stowell concluded that the dead person had suffered a broken neck.

The laminal spurs on the thoracic vertebrae – projections from the main back bone – were very small. This fact helped Stowell to establish the dead man's age, for the growth of the laminal spurs with age is measurable; he had died in about his eighteenth year. The age factor was also backed up by the un-closed sutures, or bone joins, of the skull vault.

Stowell then examined the forearm bones. The left radius had been broken in at least four places, while the ulna showed the beginning of a transverse fracture. On the basis of the *Life of St Oswald* report and these bones, Stowell concluded that the left forearm had been twisted inwards with great force.

Probably the most exciting of all was the left thigh bone, which had also suffered a greenstick fracture, a form of breakage which, as has already been noted, rarely occurs in the bones of persons older than the late 'teens. According to the *Life of St Oswald* the King's body had been forced backwards over the saddle cantle and then dragged along the ground by its left foot. Stowell had previously conducted a post-mortem on a boy apprentice who had been dragged along the ground, feet up-wards, by the driving belt of a lathe, and who had sustained precisely the same type of fracture. The left lower leg bone, the tibia, had also been broken in a greenstick fashion, and this, too, tallied with the fall which Edward was said to have undergone.

Finally, Stowell examined the right shoulderblade, the right humerus, and the right haunch bone, all of which were broken, consistent with the body falling from the saddle to strike the ground on its right side – the force being taken by the shoulder, elbow and protuberant part of the hip.

Stowell wrote in his report that the bones were those of a male of the age of King Edward, and that they showed a 'concaten-ation of fractures which precisely fit the story of the murder . . . the attack on the left upper limb, the drawing of the body to the right . . .'. He could not suggest 'any other series of violences' which could have produced the same results.

In conclusion he stated: 'I cannot escape the conviction that, on historical, anatomical, and surgical grounds, beyond reason-able doubt we have the bones of Saint Edward, King and Martyr.'

Stowell was to have many ordinary triumphs in the course of his career, which ended with his death in the early 1970s; his sensational though unproven theory that Queen Victoria's son the Duke of Clarence performed the 'Jack the Ripper' murders received wide circulation in Britain and America in the year immediately preceding his death. But no mere near-contemporary murder ever gave him the satisfaction he gained from solving the mystery of the Shaftesbury Abbey relics. Perhaps there is a moral to be drawn somewhere from the four 'historic' cases of forensic analysis outlined here: though its horror and brutality fade over the years, murder, reduced literally to its bare bones, nevertheless retains a fascination induced by no other facet of human activity.

# Chapter Thirteen
# Forensic science and the future

*If you've got a nice fresh corpse, fetch him out!*

Mark Twain, *Innocents Abroad*

In 1832, the Texas politician and cattleman Stephen F. Austin advertised for ten 'tough but honest' men, who should also be superb marksmen and expert riders, to protect the lives and property of settlers against marauding Indians and cattle-thieves. The men chosen were appointed police constables and by October 1835 they had grown in number and become so successful that they were commissioned as the first 'official' law enforcement body of the new Texas community, which was then beginning to press for independence from Mexico, under the title 'Texas Rangers'.

During the next ten years they combined their duties as lawmen with those of light cavalry during the Mexican War of Independence and were so ferocious and skilful that their opponents named them *Los Diablos Tejanos* – 'The Texas Devils'. With the sovereignty of the new state established they returned again to peace-keeping, a task which involved subduing the fiery Lipan Apaches. The Rangers still treasure an oft-quoted remark made by a chief of this tribe, Flacco, who had become a scout for Ranger Captain Jack Hayes's troop.

'Me and Red Wing,' he said, 'not afraid to go to hell together. Captain Jack not afraid to go to hell by himself.'

All this, although stirring historical stuff, might seem at first sight to have little to do with modern police work, and yet the modern Texas Rangers who sprang from these unsophisticated roots have flowered into what is arguably the most up-to-date law enforcement agency in the world. Today they operate as part of the Texas Department of Public Safety, and their own forensic science laboratory at Austin ranks second only in the United States to that of the Federal Bureau of Investigation in Washington. But further than this they have a unique distinction in police terms; each man of the force is still required to be a crack-shot with hand gun and carbine, and to be a top rider – he maintains his own horse which travels behind his car in a horsebox, ready for use in otherwise inaccessible areas – but before he receives his badge he must also pass examinations in every aspect of scientific policework. The back of every Texas Ranger's station wagon contains a mini-forensic laboratory, so that its crew can lift, photograph and process fingerprints, make rudimentary tests for the presence of blood, suspected poisons and so forth, and carry out ballistic comparisons on the spot. The area covered by Texas is vast – it is the second largest state in the Union, amounting to almost 576,000 square miles – and the incidence of crime is relatively large compared with the population of under 11 millions, an equation which makes speedy crime detection imperative. Thus, the thinking behind the system is straightforward enough. A Ranger is called to the scene of a suspected murder in a relatively inaccessible part of his territory. He does his police examination work first – tracing and taking statements from witnesses, checking the movements and habits of the deceased, inquiring after motive, and so on. But almost simultaneously he begins the tasks normally left to a forensic examiner – packeting and labelling clues, taking the temperature of the body, measuring aspects of the murder scene, dusting and lifting fingerprints where necessary. If he has paramedical training – and many Rangers take this voluntary course – he will examine and make notes of external signs of violence on the body, and where feasible will make his blood, hair and ballistics tests. The results are then communicated via radio-telephone to the main forensic laboratory at Austin, which houses, among other things, computer banks of fingerprints, gun specifications and the other basics of scientific crime fighting.

While the laboratory analyses the individual Rangers' findings from the field and begins its own wider investigation into the crime, the 'lone Ranger' metaphorically hitches up his gun belt and sets about the last stage of his task – hunting down his man.

Since the inception of this unique system in the early 1960s the Texas Rangers have been justifiably proud of the results they have obtained; some argue that apart from anything else the sheer propaganda value of having a potential criminal know that not only will he be hunted by a 'Texas Devil' but one with all the powers of modern forensic science in his pocket, as it were, is a powerful deterrent. To a much more limited extent other police forces charged with maintaining law and order over vast and relatively sparsely populated areas – the Royal Canadian Mounted Police for instance – have experimented with the system with varying results. So the obvious question asked by criminologists is – could the Texas Ranger system eventually become standard for urban police forces until every officer, at least every criminal investigation officer, becomes his own forensic expert?

The simple answer seems to be no. A senior British police officer who has studied American police methods explained:

The Rangers, because of their reputation, are an elite force and have no shortage of potential members – often their candidates are college graduates. And Texas is a rich state: its law enforcement people are paid well. Most urban forces, on the other hand, both in the United States and Europe, are understaffed and underpaid. At the moment, quite honestly, we cannot hope to attract the same standard of educated men to carry out this highly complicated work. We take the best of our men and we put them into the criminal investigation departments, where their principal duties are the detection and solution of crime. Each man has the benefit of a back-up service: telephone operators, civilian typists, car maintenance people and the rest.

Mobile crime laboratories are used as a matter of course today when a serious crime has been committed in a rural area, but these are staffed by trained forensic scientists from the nearest laboratories.

In fact, the evidence of scientists is becoming increasingly important as juries become more and more reluctant to convict on the evidence of police officers alone or on the unsupported testimony of identification evidence. Even the tried and tested fingerprint system has been called into question, which has led the experts to delve into even more esoteric fields in order to prove or disprove a particular case.

The relatively youthful discipline of psychology is one which is playing a greater role in the capture of criminals – particularly the psychopathic killer and the politically motivated criminal. In

America, most medical examiners have a trained forensic psychologist to whom they can turn, and the psychologist is often called in on even the more mundane cases – those concerning hit and run drivers for instance. A psychologist comments:

Most hit and run killers are obviously not habitual murderers. They make a mistake, knock someone down, panic and flee. Each case is dealt with in regard to its individual aspects, but in an 'average' case we might advise the police to prey on the man's guilty conscience, appealing through the media to his better nature – and that of any relatives who may know his secret – in order to get him give himself up. This is a huge over-simplification, for human reactions are of course vastly complex and differ widely from situation to situation, individual to individual. But basically we study what evidence there is and try and work out a pattern of possible behaviour.

The same thing applies to a killer who establishes a 'pattern' over a series of similar crimes. It is a truism to say that the 'Jack the Ripper' type slayer who preys on a particular type of individual will go on killing compulsively until he is either caught or, as often happens, kills himself. Such a split personality presents difficulties on the one hand, for his conscious mind may completely obliterate traces of each crime until the next urge comes upon him, and because his type of murderer is notoriously cunning in covering up his tracks. On the other hand the sheer regularity of his modus operandi may give a vital clue.

The science of statistics is also being increasingly called into forensic investigation. Since the early 1970s Dr J. W. Bracket Jnr, a leading toxicologist and Instructor in Physical Evidence at the City College Forensic Department, San Francisco, has been computerizing data on striae – the marks made by guns on bullets, and by tools used to force tills and cashboxes – in order to produce a 'ready reckoner' system for presentation to juries. The problem he has set out to solve is a highly complex one which has come about only during the past 30 years, as the standard of microscopy has become more and more advanced.

As we have seen, a rifled gun barrel leaves marks on the bullet ejected from it which are termed striae. Similarly, a chisel used to cut through wood, or a screw driver used to prize off a lock, may slip on the metal surface and leave its own striae.

While high-powered modern comparison microscopes leave little doubt that two bullets fired from the same gun have almost identical markings, the same cannot be said for striae caused by house or safe breaking tools. They may look the same, even under normal magnification, but in recent years microscopists have clashed in court as to their similarity under high power magnification. Bracket decided to investigate the problem mathematically.

First he produced tool or weapon marks in wax, plastic and other materials so that the striae could be seen. Then, using gigantic reproductions of the marks, he considered each striation as an element of a set of striae, representing a position only in two dimensional space between neighbouring elements. The position was then quantized, that is, expressed as a whole number of unit distances away from each neighbour. What Bracket terms 'geometric', 'number based', and 'outcome' models of the sets of striae were produced, and from them enormously complex graphs showing up their 'match' and 'non match' characteristics. An interim report states:

The mathematics of all these findings are currently being computerised and the results should be that, out of all this apparent confusion, police and juries will have a simple but precise range of forensic probabilities to consider, instead of such baffling propositions as, to paraphrase the old tag: 'it's a hundred percent certain she fell, and a fifty-fifty chance she was pushed'.

Dr Bracket's involved experiments are, in fact, simply an extreme extension of the age old problem which faced such pioneers as Vidocq and Bertillon – identification. And in fact, work in the field of identification, both of suspected criminals and potential ones, goes on all the time. Sometimes the theories verge on the ridiculous. It has been suggested – and most forensic pathologists would guess that the suggestion has at least a basis fact – that the markings of the human lips, for instance, are as individual as those of fingerprints or, to take a more extreme example, that each individual's stomach lining differs from that of his neighbour's.

Unfortunately the problem with such propositions is an obvious one: how do you classify such data to be of use in criminal identification? To the credit of experimental forensic science, new methods of identification continue to be tested, however, and perhaps the most exciting system perfected over the past decade has been that of voiceprinting.

Ever since the early days of the cylinder phonograph, scientists have realized that the sound of a voice can be translated into physical terms – the grooves on a record being a simple example. In the early 1960s, an experimental engineer named L. G. Kersta of the Bell Telephone Company proposed the voiceprint as a new method of forensic identification.

Mr Kersta knew that the 'articulators' – the lips, teeth, palate and tongue – are just one group of factors controlling the tonal quality of speech. Mouth, nose and throat cavities also have a decisive effect, but the overriding factor is the unconscious muscular control of all these, which produces speech patterns of varying frequencies and of characteristic timbre. The breakthrough in Mr Kersta's research came when he realized that an electronic sound analyser could detect and record frequency characteristics and harmonics – all uniquely individual – due to fundamentals of the voice cavities, and the subconscious control in every individual of his own articulators. To prove his point to himself, the engineer made recordings of 50,000 different voices, many of them apparently 'similar'. In fact all showed great differences on the cathode ray screen. He even employed professional mimics for his trials, asking them to record imitations of individuals, and then comparing the results with recordings of the person imitated. The results on graph and screen were again greatly dissimilar.

In April 1966, Kersta felt ready to demonstrate his techniques before a jury; through no fault of his own he failed to obtain a conviction. A New Rochelle police officer was brought to trial at Westchester County Court on an unusual charge of perjury. The allegation was that he had warned a professional gambler of an impending police raid; the District Attorney had suspected that such a tip-off would be made, and had had the officer's phone tapped and allowed Kersta and his technicians to set up their recording equipment. Later, with the suspect's permission, the prints were compared with open microphone prints, and both Kersta and the DA considered them to be identical.

In the witness box, Kersta demonstrated examples of his voice test. Though impressed, the defence attorney challenged the legal, rather than technical, competence of the witness, and the judge ruled that the jury must decide on the point. The jury disagreed, and due to the complex nature of United States law the case reached the Supreme Court, which ruled that the New York state law which had permitted the phone-tapping – not the voice printing – was unconstitutional. This meant that none of the telephone evidence could be allowed and the case was dismissed.

Kersta, however, had made an impression in forensic circles and set up his own company, Voiceprint Laboratories, under licence from the Bell Telephone Company. The news spread to Europe and, rather unfairly for Kersta, the first legal vindication of his technique came at Winchester petty sessional court in November 1967, when a man was charged with making obscene telephone calls. There was no question of the legality of the police tapping the phone involved, nor of the voiceprint technique, and recordings were made on high fidelity audio tape. These were frequency-analysed at Leeds University and the results convinced the magistrates, who convicted and fined the defendant. It was perhaps the biggest step forward for forensic science since the acceptance of fingerprints by Scotland Yard, and yet it made few headlines.

It was Kersta himself, appropriately enough, who conducted the tests which first made voiceprints world-wide news. In 1967, at the time of the Watts riots, a CBS TV news interviewer named Bill Stout interviewed a number of black youths in the thick of the fighting. One of them turned his back to the camera so that his face could not be seen and boasted of having been involved in the burning of several Los Angeles shops. After the broadcast, police tracked down an 18-year-old Negro youth named Edward Lee King, who naturally denied the charge. However, he was held in custody pending prosecution on a narcotics charge.

Kersta now analysed the soundtrack of Bill Stout's film, and compared it with voiceprints which he was able to obtain from the imprisoned King. The two tallied exactly. This time the jury accepted the evidence of voiceprints at the end of the seven-week long arson trial, and King was convicted and jailed. As a result two legal technicalities arose, involving the privilege against self-incrimination, and the right of a defendant to refuse to make a print for comparison. Two rulings, one by the State of New Jersey Superior Court, and the other by the United States Supreme Court, ruled that a defendant had no right to refuse tape recordings or voiceprinting, and that the right of protection against self-incrimination did not apply. Since then, Kersta's techniques have been used successfully both in the United States and elsewhere.

A rather more mundane – but arguably more vital – system of identification perfected by the FBI Sex Crimes Investigation department in the early 1970s, which operates on a digital code principle rather similar to that used by Alphonse Bertillon, has revolutionized the fight against sex offenders in recent years. It works in conjunction with the British forensic scientist Jacques Penry's invention, patented in 1971 and known as the Penry Facial Identification Technique, or 'Photo-fit'.

Basically, offenders convicted of sexual crime are classified under seven digits ranging from one to seven, consisting of the categories: white, negro, other, age, height, build, hair. Then comes a further eleven sub-categories of noticeable peculiarities: limp or gait; eye-glasses; visible scars, crooked, deformed or missing limbs; tattoos; speech; moustache or beard; mentality retarded; ears, hearing defects; teeth, mouth: complexion, moles; and finally left-handed.

Then comes the classification of their sexual tendencies, comprising almost forty categories of astonishing variety. These range from such 'normal' categories as incest, rape and sodomy, through to such esoteric items as 'car exposers', 'impersonating with intent to commit offence (police, doctor, minister)', 'frotteurs, rubbers and hair offences', 'ladies' underwear involvement (stealing and wearing)' and 'setting fires in the course of a sexual act'. There are a whole range of 'molesters' including 'midtown molesters (department stores and cinemas)', 'downtown molesters (ramp garages and parking lots)' and park, playing ground, nurses' home, girls' dormitory, bus, cab, and university area molesters.

Bizarre as the list seems, linked as it is with the sexual offenders' computer at the FBI forensic laboratory and backed up by the Photo-fit team, the classification technique has resulted in hundreds of prompt captures and convictions since its inception. The whole set-up is further aided by the Habitual Sexual Offenders Law, first enacted in Ohio in 1963 and since codified across the country. This requires any person convicted more than twice of a sexual offence to register with the local law enforcement agency before staying in one county for more than 30 days. In the event of a particular type of crime taking place, the FBI then checks on the whereabouts of the likely suspects through this system, in conjunction with its own computerized data.

But important as all these innovations – along with others in the earliest experimental stages – are, it is the small-scale up-dating of established techniques which inches forensic science forward on a workday plane. The modern computer, for instance, is employed at all levels. One toxicologist explained his use of the machine:

I use the thing for prognosis. If I am faced, say, with a chemical end-product which could have come about due to a combination of factors, I feed all the possibilities into the computer until it comes up with a probability. Only then do I begin to test that probability at the bench in the old-fashioned way. The computer saves an awful lot of time.

Time has always been of the essence in scientific crime fighting, so that the modern forensic science laboratory is a masterpiece of efficiency. The staff at one of Europe's most up-to-date crime laboratories, that at Wetherby in Yorkshire, take a quiet pride in their growing reputation, and yet insist that they are simply doing what all their overseas colleagues are also achieving – making an ever more sophisticated inroad into the world of the lawbreaker.

The North Eastern Forensic Laboratory, to give it its Home Office title, was opened in April 1977, to replace the two antiquated establishments at Harrogate and Newcastle. It cost a total of £1,600,000, of which about £500,000 was spent on scientific equipment. With these tools, the sixty plus staff of scientists and technicians under the directorship of Peter Cobb, formerly head of Harrogate laboratory, serve the police forces of seven counties, the principal ones being those in Yorkshire and Humberside.

Set in the semi-rural surroundings near Wetherby's famous race course, the laboratory buildings look rather like a light industrial plant, and are, in fact, deceptively large. The whole of the Nottingham laboratory, one of the oldest in use and perched on the top floor of Nottingham police station could, it is said, be accommodated in just one of Wetherby's workshops. Basically the complex is split into three wings, specializing in biology, chemistry, and toxicology, but it also contains a photographic section, conference and lecture rooms, a large and well equipped vehicle examination garage and a mortuary section, for though autopsies are not normally carried out here, the bodies of more baffling cases of suicide or murder are often re-examined on the premises.

The biology section concerns itself with offences against the person – murder, rape, wounding – as well as the examination of hair and fibres. The central section of the biology department is known as the 'search room' where samples are obtained for testing and identification. The priorities of the search room are fixed by the time taken by various samples to deteriorate; swabs of semen and saliva, for instance, must be tested as soon as possible because of deterioration, while a little more time can be taken with blood samples. Hair and fibres come last in the list, chronologically speaking, but are treated with the same importance.

A bloodstain of less than half an inch can be tested quickly to see if it is human or animal, and if it is the latter its origin can be traced rapidly. Saliva and semen can also be classified in a way which narrows down their origin to less than ten percent of the population.

It is possible to identify particles of fibre less than one millimetre long and, if a man is picked up by the police two days after a crime, it is more than possible he has some particle on his clothes that may link him with the crime. When the suspect's clothes are brought to the search room, possible samples are 'lifted' with a fairly mundane looking adhesive roller. Any threads and hairs are then examined using a range of microscopes and a series of light filtering techniques.

The toxicology department, staffed by 14 scientists, is possibly the hardest pressed section, in terms of cases handled. In the first years of its existence, the laboratory handled over 15,000 cases and no less than two thirds of these were drunken driving matters. To ease pressure, alcohol levels in blood samples taken after the offence are now tested by an automatic process, and if the readings hover around the legal limit a total of four further tests may be made. Each test takes only four minutes in one of the bank of analysers with an automatic print out.

As well as drunken driving cases, the toxicology department also deals, of course, with poisons and drug abuse – a field which has increased greatly during the last decade. Containers of cannabis plants, samples of hashish, LSD tablets and other drugs line the shelves of the drug section, where technicians identify each sample brought in by police. In most cases, the experts can tell readily from what source and what part of the world the drug has originated. The increased volume of work, said a spokesman, is largely due to the number of police prosecutions in recent years, and the increased number of officers assigned to drug offences.

The toxicology department also work side by side with the chemistry and biology sections in that most unpleasant of crime laboratory tasks, the analysis of stomach contents, to determine time and cause of death. Sections of human tissue are also examined for fuller reports after the regular autopsy.

The chemistry department deals largely with offences against property. Again the bulk of work concerns traffic accidents. In these cases, a splinter of paint or a shard of glass can be of vital importance. Paint flakes are placed on edge under a microscope so that the various layers can be determined; these are then compared with colour charts and individual painting processes supplied by the world's car manufacturers and kept on file, so that first a make, then a year, can be identified, and later matched to the vehicle. Items like car trims and hub caps are kept in a special collection at the Home Office's central laboratory at

Aldermaston, and a telephonic link to the computers there keeps Wetherby investigators up to the minute.

Similarly, glass fragments at the scene of a crime can be identified and matched using an instrument called a hot stage microscope. Under this the glass is heated to a temperature where its refractive index can be read, and the results are fed to the Aldermaston computers, which will certainly tell how common the glass is and usually the name of the manufacturer. Painstaking manual work, however, is also called for when dealing with glass. Often the department will reconstruct, jig-saw like, a whole headlight from shattered portions found at the scene of an accident, and on at least one occasion, where a window had been broken at the scene of a crime and the glass swept up before the significance of the breakage was noticed, Wetherby scientists had an even tougher assignment on their hands. The entire window was reconstructed, piece by piece – including even tiny fragments – to show whether the broken pane had fallen inwards or outwards. Again, a beer bottle used in a violent murder assault was reconstructed and matched against a plaster cast of the victim's skull to show how and where the blow had landed.

Perhaps the pride of the chemistry department is one of the newest pieces of scientific equipment, a laser microspectral analyser. This uses a small laser beam to burn a minute crater in metal or other material and then analyses the vapour given off. By this means it is possible to tell exactly what components are present in the substance.

Gas chromatography is used, among other applications, to test materials from fires where arson is suspected, by extracting a sample of vapour from re-heated debris from the scene; the instrument separates and identifies the ingredients present. If gasoline or kerosene is present, the probability of arson is high. However, the human element often remains invaluable, here as in other fields of criminal science. On one occasion after a house had been razed by fire, police, insurance, and forensic science investigators visited the site and after a careful check deduced that the blaze had been a result of an accident. On the way out, however, one of the forensic examiners noticed a portion of charred doormat, picked it up and, out of idle curiosity, sniffed it. He thought he detected a lingering whiff of gasolene, and the gas chromatograph proved him correct. A petrol bomb had been pushed through the front door, but the blaze had spread and caused most damage further inside the house, drawing the attention of the investigators away from the true cause.

Currently, Britain spends upwards of £5,000,000 on the Home Office Forensic Science Service, which is divided between Wetherby and its six fellow laboratories – at least one of them a top secret establishment – scattered throughout England and Wales. All crime laboratory activity is collated and administered through the central laboratory at Aldermaston, housed in the former Atomic Research Centre there.

Information from all the regional laboratories is collated and computerized and constant analysis of the details results in learned papers which are circularized in Britain and abroad, over 27,000 having been written in the past decade. In toxicology alone, Aldermaston scientists have made strides which would have been unthinkable 20 years ago, for today the amount of blood needed for drug or poison analysis may be no more than .0000000001 grams. A process known as high pressure liquid chromatography can detect tiny traces of substances such as LSD in urine samples, while strength of dosage can be monitored by radio immunal assay technique. A new process currently 'under wraps' is said to have updated the old 'nitrate detection' system of detecting whether or not an individual has recently fired a gun or handled explosives, differentiating between, say, the nitrates deposited on the hands of cigarette smokers and those caused by discharging a revolver. And on a more mundane level, a statistical survey of 10,000 burglaries is currently being carried out to isolate common factors and bring them to police attention.

Admirable, therefore, as the Texas Rangers' 'personal forensic lab' system may be, it is with the dedication and perception of the world's forensic scientists that crime fighting in the twenty-first century will increasingly lie.

# Index

Martin Gosch and Richard Hammer
**The Luciano Testament** £1.50

America's most notorious gangster tells all ... Bribe by bribe, killing by killing, Charlie 'Lucky' Luciano came to be *capo di tutti capi*, boss of all the bosses, from Calone to Dutch Schulz and Bugsy Siegel. Companion to society women, confidant of politicians, he bought judges, union leaders, policemen to change the face of the Mafia. Told against the violent backcloth of America's underworld from the twenties to the fifties, this is the controversial story of his rise and fall.

Gerold Frank
**The Boston Strangler** £1.95

The most bizarre series of murders since Jack the Ripper; the greatest man-hunt in the annals of modern crime; Albert DeSalvo, brutal sexual psychopath, who murdered thirteen women and held a city in the icy grip of terror for eighteen hideous months.

'Tells us everything about the case ... chronologically, as it happened ... the result is completely satisfying' NEW YORKER

Gay Talese
**Thy Neighbour's Wife** £1.75

The story of how they brought sex out from behind the closed doors of the marital bedroom and made it a growth industry. Gay Talese journeys through a world of massage parlours and blue movies, topless bars and group sex ... A sensational odyssey through sexuality in our time.

'Amazingly compulsive documentary about the sexual revolution ... It cannot be put down. You can't, you mustn't miss it'
COSMOPOLITAN

'One of the best reporters in town ... a blockbuster bestseller' NOW

## James McClure
### Spike Island £1.95

'A' Division is known as 'Spike Island' in the trade – the trade being policing in that bit of Liverpool that's like a band-aid stuck over where they ripped the heart out – the toughest inner-city area in Europe.

'Shows us the truth of the policeman's job through the eyes of the men and women who actually do it ... also a book about ourselves, about the society we have created, and about the precariousness of the bridges ... over the chasm of poverty and crime' P. D. JAMES, NEW YORK TIMES

'Brilliant reportage' EVENING STANDARD

## Emlyn Williams
### Beyond Belief £1.95

The story of the Moors Murderers, Ian Brady and Myra Hindley.

'I keep remindin' myself' Superintendent Talbot said to me, 'that this isn't a tale – that it's been happening...'

'Perhaps the greatest value of this book is that it shows us that the human monsters Brady and Hindley were not one and the same, but two different kinds of monster' TIMES LITERARY SUPPLEMENT

'An appalling subject, and overpowering book' SUNDAY EXPRESS

## Selected Bestsellers

| | | | |
|---|---|---|---|
| ☐ | **Symptoms** | edited by Sigmund Stephen Miller | £2.50p |
| ☐ | **Gone with the Wind** | Margaret Mitchell | £2.95p |
| ☐ | **Robert Morley's Book of Worries** | Robert Morley | £1.50p |
| ☐ | **The Totem** | David Morrell | £1.25p |
| ☐ | **Platinum Logic** | Tony Parsons | £1.75p |
| ☐ | **The Alternative Holiday Catalogue** | edited by Harriet Peacock | £1.95p |
| ☐ | **The Pan Book of Card Games** | Hubert Phillips | £1.50p |
| ☐ | **Food for All the Family** | Magnus Pyke | £1.50p |
| ☐ | **Everything Your Doctor Would Tell You If He Had the Time** | Claire Rayner | £4.95p |
| ☐ | **Rage of Angels** | Sidney Sheldon | £1.75p |
| ☐ | **A Town Like Alice** | Nevil Shute | £1.50p |
| ☐ | **Just Off for the Weekend** | John Slater | £2.50p |
| ☐ | **A Falcon Flies** | Wilbur Smith | £1.95p |
| ☐ | **The Deep Well at Noon** | Jessica Stirling | £1.75p |
| ☐ | **The Eighth Dwarf** | Ross Thomas | £1.25p |
| ☐ | **The Music Makers** | E. V. Thompson | £1.50p |
| ☐ | **The Third Wave** | Alvin Toffler | £1.95p |
| ☐ | **The Flier's Handbook** | | £4.95p |

All these books are available at your local bookshop or newsagent, or can be ordered direct from the publisher. Indicate the number of copies required and fill in the form below

4

Name _____
(block letters please)

Address _____

_____

Send to Pan Books (CS Department), Cavaye Place, London SW10 9PG
Please enclose remittance to the value of the cover price plus :
35p for the first book plus 15p per copy for each additional book ordered
to a maximum charge of £1.25 to cover postage and packing
Applicable only in the UK

While every effort is made to keep prices low, it is sometimes necessary to increase prices at short notice. Pan Books reserve the right to show on covers and charge new retail prices which may differ from those advertised in the text or elsewhere